How to Succeed in Writing a Book

Ruth Chambers, Gill Wakley,
Gillian Nineham and Gregory Moxon
with Michele Topham

Radcliffe Publishing
Oxford • Seattle

Radcliffe Publishing Ltd
18 Marcham Road
Abingdon
Oxon OX14 1AA
United Kingdom

www.radcliffe-oxford.com
Electronic catalogue and worldwide online ordering facility.

———————————————————————————

British Library Cataloguing in Publication Data

A catalogue record for this book is available from the British Library.

ISBN-10: 1 84619 039 8
ISBN-13: 978 1 84619 039 1

Typeset by Anne Joshua & Associates, Oxford
Printed and bound by TJ International Ltd, Padstow, Cornwall

Contents

Preface iv
About the authors v

1 Why write a book?
   Ruth Chambers 1

2 When and what to write
   Ruth Chambers and Gill Wakley 13

3 In what capacity will you be writing?
   Ruth Chambers 25

4 How to write a convincing book proposal
   Ruth Chambers 37

5 Choosing a publisher
   Gill Wakley 49

6 Having a literary agent
   Michele Topham 57

7 Writing the book
   Gill Wakley 63

8 Style
   Gill Wakley 75

9 The publisher's side: editorial and production
   Gill Nineham 91

10 The publisher's side: finance, marketing and promotion
   Gregory Moxon 103

11 Improving your writing technique
   Ruth Chambers 113

Index 119

Preface

This is a 'how to do it' book for anyone considering writing a book. It is mainly directed at people in the health and social care sectors, to help them start. It helps inexperienced or frustrated authors realise where they may be going wrong. They can learn how to improve their approach to writing so that their books can be published.

Learn how to write to be understood. Pick up tips from the five authors of this book who have all been in the writing and publishing business for a long time. Although the book focuses on writing for health and social care, most of the information and guidance about getting published can be transferred to any kind of book or publication.

Ruth Chambers
September 2006

About the authors

Ruth Chambers
Ruth has been a GP for more than 20 years and is currently the Director of Postgraduate GP Education at West Midlands Deanery and Professor of Primary Care at Staffordshire University. She has written more than 50 books over the last seven years with three publishers – mainly for health professionals, but some for the general public. She has also written and published innumerable articles, mainly about healthcare, in peer-reviewed journals and the popular medical press, and has a health column in her local evening newspaper.

Gill Wakley
Gill started in general practice in 1966, but transferred to community medicine shortly afterwards and then into public health. A desire for increased contact with patients caused a move back into general practice, together with community gynaecology, in 1978. She combined the two, in varying amounts, together with some academic primary care, until her recent retirement. Throughout she has been heavily involved in learning and teaching. She has written, or contributed to, a large number of books on a variety of primary care subjects. She is an advisory editor for the *Journal of Family Planning and Reproductive Medicine*, and keeps a keen eye on the style and content of the journal. She is enthusiastic about trying to raise the standard of writing by medics and allied professionals.

Gillian Nineham
Gill is Editorial Director of Radcliffe Publishing, a role she has held almost since the company was established in 1987. She is responsible for the majority of commissioning activity and new project development at Radcliffe, and she works closely with authors and editors, as well as with organisations with which the company collaborates.

Before joining the company she worked for a small travel publisher, and subsequently spent a short time in the marketing department of Blackwell Science and then as a project developer and producer in film and video production.

Gregory Moxon
Gregory has worked in publishing for 25 years. He has specialised in business development, sales and marketing across various media, including art publishing, television, video and computer games, as well as books. After roles at companies including Granada Television and Octopus Books, he joined Radcliffe in 1995 as its first Head of Marketing. Here he leads the marketing team, working closely with authors, commercial customers and partner organisations to develop and promote Radcliffe's publications in print and electronic formats.

Michele Topham

Michele has been working for literary agencies since 1984 and is now with the Felicity Bryan Literary Agency. Founded in 1988, the agency represents a wide variety of distinguished authors of adult non-fiction, fiction and children's literature. Based in Oxford, the agency sells book rights throughout the world and works closely with a number of film and TV agents. Michele's work experience includes liaising with authors, editorial work, rights and contracts, and royalty accounts.

Chapter 1

Why write a book?

Ruth Chambers

There are a myriad reasons to tempt you into becoming an author. This is especially true if writing a book is a cherished dream that you have held for years – even most of your life.

It can be frustrating to find that there is no useful book when you are training or teaching others. You might be producing handouts and designing interactive work programmes to fill that gap for your students or trainees. Then it is only a few more steps to putting together a book proposal, drawing on the preparatory work of your teaching.

You might consider that the standard texts that underpin your teaching or training could be much improved or progressed in thinking. That might fuel you to write a book yourself and improve the standard of textbooks available in the area. You may have been running courses on a subject in which you are an expert. You have written course notes and would like to expand them into the book you think would best inform and assist your students. You may have been irritated by the lack of usefulness of textbooks on a subject you know well, and feel that you could do much better yourself.

On the other hand, you may not be in a teaching or training position, but wish to convey the essence of your experience as a health or social care professional or manager. This might be relevant to anyone working in hospital or community healthcare, or in social care. You might be a student on a course, reading the book out of interest or for your professional development. You may feel dismayed by the way that health or social care is planned or delivered. You feel that you can improve the way in which people do things, with your guidance or by developing and relaying case studies.

Perhaps someone else has suggested that you could write a good book on a subject, or has invited you to become a co-author. But do take care. You may have been encouraged by the maxim that 'everyone has a book inside them' to believe that you, too, have the talent to write a book, certain that your best-seller is just waiting to burst out if you only had the time to write it. The above saying probably refers to the stories people have to tell that have evolved from their experiences, rather than the type of book you might be writing for health or social care students or professionals that is 'work related.' So you might not be receptive to the cautions here against writing a reasoned book and dismiss the drawbacks and warnings as applying to other people – not you.

You will have more idea of the magnitude of the task that you are embarking on in writing a book if you already write articles for the popular press, or academic papers for professional journals or detailed reports as an integral part of your day job. If you are used to these kinds of publications, you should have a

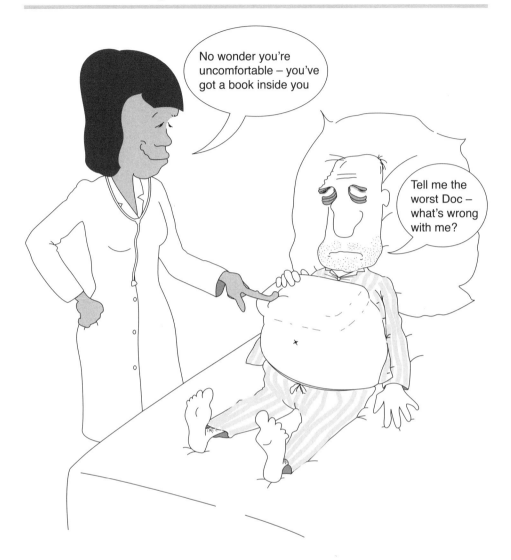

keen understanding of the time and effort spent in preparing to write – gathering material, crafting your 'writing project' for a particular readership, and liaising with a potential publisher or commissioning editor. And that is when you are on a smooth track moving forward and before you even start the hard work. If you are a complete novice with a dream, then try to break the spell you are under and chat to experienced writers, or register for an introductory writing course so that you can weigh the pros and cons of proceeding to write a book.

One of the best ways to ensure that you complete the manuscript you start, and that it serves its purpose, is to be certain of why you are going to write the book in the first place. It may be that for some reason you are expected or required to write a book as part of your role. You may want to establish yourself as an authority or to maintain your expert profile in a particular field. You may want to share what you know or leave a legacy for others to read. You might think that you can make some money from sales of your publications that were previously restricted to being in-house. The book could be a 'loss leader', not a commercial success but advertising other services that you provide. It could be one or all of these things, or you might have other motivators. If you are certain about what is motivating you to write the book, then if or when the going gets tough, you can revisit your reason(s) for writing to encourage yourself to keep going. And you can check out your progress against those motivators. For instance, if you are writing the book to make money, you will want to get away with as short a manuscript as possible.

Read and heed the warnings throughout this book. Absorb the guidance we are offering that is intended to eliminate any false starts and accelerate your writing project. Find ways to minimise the work or responsibility of writing a book – for example, by teaming up with other writers, or updating other published work with the original authors for a new edition.

What are you getting into?

Box 1.1 gives you an idea of the time that writing a book will take you. The figures in the Box are just a guess relating to the time that an experienced author would take to write a book of, say, 50,000 words (to help you gauge what that looks like, the bulk of this book minus the introductory pages and indexing is approximately 45,000 words). You'll see that we have put the number of hours in a writing day as being 10 hours, not the standard 7.5–8.0 hours. This is because when you are absorbed in writing, you may find that you generally keep going until you finish a section, postponing meals or other activities. Because few people can timetable writing a book into their working day, most authors cram their writing into any spare time they have available, so once they've got the opportunity to write they keep going, on and on, and on . . .

Box 1.1 Guesstimate of minimum time for an experienced solo author to write a book of 50,000 words, once the book proposal is agreed

Phase 1: Prepare to write

Maybe 5 days for research and background information, literature search, library visits and requests.

Maybe 2 days to collate information already in your possession – in files, previous and current work.

Subtotal	7 days

Phase 2: Prepare and submit manuscript

Say 5,000 words per 10-hour day (draft manuscript).

First-draft manuscript	10 days (100 hours)
Editing and revision to second-draft manuscript	3 days
Final revision in response to others' critique, and updating manuscript → submit manuscript	2 days
Subtotal	15 days

Phase 3: Book promotion and final amendments

Complete book promotion questionnaire	3 hours
Respond to editor queries	7 hours
Proofread copy-edited manuscript and correct errors	1 day
Subtotal	2 days
Total	24 days (10-hour days)

Then you need to realise what else you could be doing instead. How can you justify the 24 days or 240 hours – or maybe twice that amount of time if you are inexperienced as a writer, or in the field about which you are writing? Box 1.2 gives you some ideas about what else you could be doing instead – attending and speaking at conferences if you're an academic, giving lectures or running workshops, speaking on the radio, planning for and undertaking research or doing lots and lots of health, leisure or family activities. You will be able to make a mental calculation to weigh up your alternative options in this way.

Box 1.2 What else can you do with 24 days instead of writing a book?

1 If you are an academic or conference buff you could travel to and attend up to ten national or international conferences.
2 If you want to share your ideas and thinking, you could give presentations, radio discussions or lectures, or run workshops instead. You could prepare for and deliver six presentations at national conferences and run a dozen workshops and lectures, and still have time for networking.
3 If you are a researcher, you might write a research proposal, prepare drafts of a research ethics submission, identify funding and research or support colleagues in doing so, and start to action the research protocol.

4   If you are overworked already, and the writing of the book is destined for your weekends, nights and early mornings, you could just use these 24 'days' and reflection time to do sports and exercise, go on family outings, play games with the kids or spend time with your partner or seeking a new partner.

Why write? You know a lot and want to share it

You could be new in post, having moved in from outside the health or social care setting and seeing opportunities to generalise your experience and expertise from another public or private sector organisation to the health or social care setting. Alternatively, you may have worked in the health or social care setting for a long time and taken a career step to other employment or set up as an independent consultant, like Roy in Box 1.3. Then you will be able to reflect back on how well things were working and could be improved by adopting the different ways of working in your new organisation or those workplaces where you are acting as consultant. It could even be that by looking in at health and social care from the outside you understand how well things are going, and your book is about valuing and treasuring current systems or working lives. Whatever your particular situation described here, you are in a really good position to compare what is happening with what is possible, and to help others to realise how to close that gap – to improve the way things or people work. This will build on your bank of knowledge and transferable skills.

Box 1.3

Roy was a senior manager in the National Health Service (NHS) in the UK for many years. He became an independent consultant with a portfolio career that included an attachment to a university health policy centre. His books capture the essence of the systems and processes that the NHS needs to adopt in new areas of development or change, to help readers to progress and improve the ways of working in their teams and organisations.

Another possible scenario is that you are nearing retirement or at the end of a section in your career, and you want to leave a 'legacy' of what you have learned on the job, to make it easier for those who come after you, like Lizzie in Box 1.4.

Box 1.4

Lizzie was a fifth-year medical student when she agreed to accept a commission from a publisher to co-write a 'survival guide for medical students.' She joined other students in the writing team who brought in their different backgrounds, pooling their experiences of the difficulties, challenges and opportunities that arose from the time when they were accepted to medical school until they had successfully exited it.

Why write a book? You write articles and want to progress

Writing articles or columns for newspapers or journals is much easier than writing a book. The former kind of writing requires short bursts of energy around a particular topic with maybe three or four key points. Your article might be composed of straight text or questions and answers, which compared with a book is fairly short and focused, and your effort is not sustained. You will probably get paid for your articles, too, which on a payment per word count far exceeds what you might expect to receive from royalties or a commission for most non-fiction, professional books.

Having said that, if you are experienced at writing articles, you will have a good idea of the magnitude of the task that you face in writing a book. You will probably already have developed your writing style and systems. You will have become quicker and slicker at writing than when you set out. You will have established your ways for gathering ideas, maybe carrying a notebook with you to jot down ideas when you are out and about, or keeping that fluorescent pen by your bedside for the scintillating thoughts that come to you there. You may already be known as a writer, and that should make it easier for you to get your book proposal accepted by a publisher, who will be more sure of your success as a book writer – and that people will buy your book – like Ruth in Box 1.5.

Box 1.5

Ruth wrote articles on clinical and non-clinical topics for newspapers destined for general practitioners for a couple of years. She was always aware of their short shelf-life, and that many of the varied members of the primary care team did not read the articles, because of the limited circulation of the newspapers in which they were published. A chance meeting with a publisher stimulated her to compile a book proposal based on her current work in running clinical effectiveness workshops. The publisher peer-reviewed and accepted the book proposal, certain that the book would sell well as Ruth was already well known as a writer through her newspaper articles. They were right – the book is now in its fourth edition seven years later, albeit with co-authors now.[1]

Once you are a published writer, you will probably become aware of other authors. If you intend to write your book with others or edit a book rather than write a substantial number of the chapters, you will already know other writers whom you can invite to join you in the proposed book enterprise.

When it comes down to it, people generally read and later throw away newspapers and their personal copies of journals – but they will keep a book on their bookshelf (even if they don't look at it!). So you are right to want to progress from writing articles to penning a book if you want your thoughts to be captured for posterity, or at least for a few years.

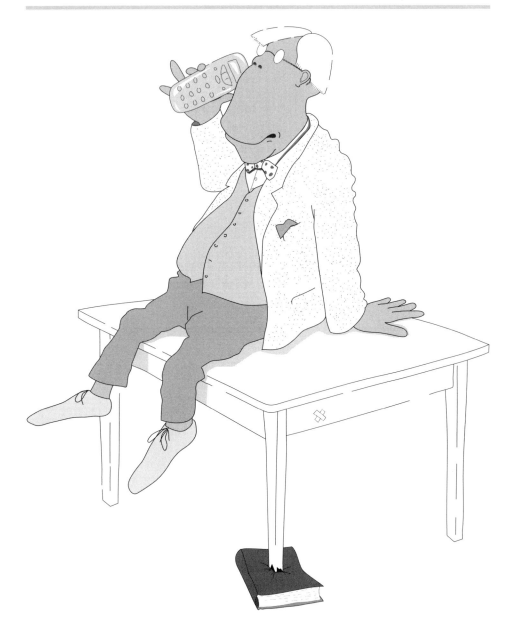

I do like your book...it's just the right depth for me.

Why write a book? Is it easier for you than talking?

If you are shy or diffident, you may find it difficult to talk to a group of other people. Your inner fears may include becoming tongue-tied or blushing self-consciously as they turn to look at you, blurting out your thinking in an incoherent way, or generally making a mess of things. This may not just be to a gathering of hundreds of people on the plenary platform of a conference, but could be at a seminar of ten or twelve people. If you have little self-confidence, even contributing in a well-phrased and authoritative way to a formal committee meeting can be daunting.

If you are a reflective kind of person and many of your ideas and beliefs are debated internally in your head, you may need time to formulate your thinking and shape it into a form that makes sense to others. So if you are of this personality type, it is difficult to join in a discussion with more extroverted individuals, as by the time you have reflected on someone else's contribution and worked on it in your head, the topic or focus of the discussion may have changed. Or you may think that the general discussion is travelling in such a simplistic way that your well-justified ideas will sound pompous or judgemental and will alienate you from others present – an especially difficult situation if you are low down in the hierarchy or experience stakes. Michael turned to writing after these kinds of struggles, as described in Box 1.6.

If these descriptions fit you, then you may find it easier to write a book than to talk without preparation or opportunity for reflection, or to address a gathering of people. This way you can take your time when formulating your thoughts, and when checking out your reasoning and beliefs with others whose opinions you value. Being the author of the book puts you on an at least level playing field with your readers, and with the peer reviewers whom journals or organisations may appoint to give their public perspectives on your eventual book. Writing a book and actually seeing your thoughts in print will also give you confidence in your ability to contribute to debates. This should then feed back to your psyche to build up your self-esteem and ability to contribute to public debates or give the presentations that you shunned initially.

Box 1.6

Michael had been a social worker, and then a team leader, who was being given more senior responsibilities. He was especially interested in the needs of disabled people and had become involved in a special interest association for disability rights. He returned home from the national meetings hating himself for not contributing to the debates. He could have said plenty but was unable to push himself to break into what he perceived as the 'inner circle.' So he started writing articles for the social care press. Another writer who was putting together a book on disability invited him to write a chapter on disability. This led to a writing friendship, and the two were soon co-writing other books together on various aspects of social care.

When you prove yourself through the concepts you express in your books, you could well attract more invitations to speak or input into local or national planning than you can cope with. So instead of pining for openings to contribute your thinking as you were in your pre-writing period, you could be prioritising and turning down the kind of invitations you could only have dreamed of before.

Why write a book? The achievement of a personal goal – you always wanted to write

Many moons ago in your schooldays, you may have had difficulty in choosing between a health or social care professional or management career track – when you selected science or arts courses at school or university. So you may have been hankering for decades to utilise your creative side that has been lying fallow while you pursued a scientific or business type of career. Now that you have so much to communicate about from your experience and expertise gained during your career, it is a good time to start writing.

Some people, like Lynne in Box 1.7, have set a personal goal of writing – articles or a book – when they have taken time out to refresh or re-energise their career, as part of a sabbatical or alongside their regular job.

Box 1.7

Lynne's best grades at school were in English language and history. She had loved writing stories from childhood, and fancied pursuing a related career such as journalism. But her parents pressured her to study science 'A'-levels with a view to taking a nursing degree, which they perceived to offer a more worthwhile and better paid career. This has paid off in the end as Lynne, as a nurse, has endless copy for writing her books, and is not competing to be published against thousands of journalists and would-be authors without healthcare experience.

Why write a book? It is expected in your role

If you are an academic or other kind of educator, as well as or instead of being a health or social care professional or manager, you will be expected to be or become a published author. To start with this may involve writing articles or research or project reports in professional publications, but as you rise up the career ladder you could well be expected or required to write a book to further establish your expert status in one or more fields. This might be part of your portfolio for a national research assessment exercise (RAE) or other quality assurance review. Although in the UK's RAE the status of a book is ranked lower than that of a published research report in a prestigious peer-reviewed journal, this is more the case for books that compile others' thinking on a subject and contain little original material from the author, or books that are more opinion based rather than underpinned by a systematic gathering of evidence.

If you are a reluctant author, forced to write because it is required or expected of you, you will have a difficult time sustaining the effort required for a single-authored book. So you may be better piggybacking on other enthusiastic authors and contributing chapters to their books.

Why write a book? A publisher asks you

You may be buzzing along in your career creating interest wherever you go. Your ideas and energy might attract the interest of a publisher on the lookout for potential authors of books that will address a gap in their range of publications. This is especially likely if your work involves new developments and is leading where national policy is likely to take the health or social care sectors. You might be on government working parties in that new area, or an adviser to your professional organisation – and so have insider knowledge and lots of insight into future difficulties and possible solutions.

Or the publisher might be from a new venture, maybe setting up in order to publish books for the general public. Then the publisher might invite you to write with them to relay your well-established professional experience in ways that the lay reader can understand.

Where the publisher is seeking an author, possibly to deliver within a short timescale, they may be prepared to agree a commission. In this case you are paid a set amount for submitting the manuscript and at publication and if the book sells more than a pre-determined number of copies, rather than receiving a share in the royalties from sales of the book. A few writers are paid to write material for projects which then form books as their regular job, like Chris in Box 1.8. Or you may act as a 'ghost' writer, revising a famous or prestigious person's material into a readable text.

Box 1.8

Chris was commissioned by a national initiative that aimed to enable ordinary people to take more care of themselves. The project paid her a set rate for the 25,000 words that she produced. This manuscript then became half of a wider book that was produced with Chris as co-author to make the material more readily available to healthcare professionals to promote to their patients.

How and why does an author keep going with their writing?

It is difficult when there are so many practical considerations and time pressures involved in putting the book together in the course of the writing and publication process. Of course, you have your everyday life to lead, too. Much of the motivation and determination to complete the writing will be derived from your reasons for doing it. An academic may need the publication in order to further their career. The book could be one of several key publications for adding to their CV to render them eligible to be short-listed for another more senior or well-paid post. It might contribute to the work undertaken for a doctorate or recognised for an honorary award. One or more of these reasons should provide the academic with the motivation to complete their writing within a specific timescale or else risk holding up their career advancement. A teacher or expert in the field might be motivated by the need or desire to get their thinking out in the public domain in order to influence the way others think about a problem or issue, and to enhance their expert status. These reasons will have an impetus, too. An author of a book for health or social care professionals might be motivated by the desire to guide others in 'how to do' some new system or procedure that has arisen from a new health or social care policy or requirement. Again, the sooner the authors complete their writing and the book is published, the more pertinent and useful it will be for the target readership that is struggling to implement the health or social care requirement or model.

Reference

1 Chambers R, Boath E, Rogers D. *Clinical Effectiveness and Clinical Governance Made Easy.* 4th ed. Oxford: Radcliffe Publishing; 2007.

Chapter 2

When and what to write

Ruth Chambers and Gill Wakley

The sooner you write a book the better, while the material is still fresh and interesting. A book goes out of date very quickly. It becomes dated as soon as you have checked the final draft and submitted the manuscript to be published. You will have a chance to update any key points in the book when you undertake the final checking of the copy-edited manuscript before it goes off for printing. So, once the book writing is under way, try to minimise the length of time you and others spend writing it, so that the task does not drag on.

Do you write as an expert or as a novice?

There are two sides to this conundrum.

As an expert

You will have plenty to write about and will give your views with the authority of your long experience and established expertise.

You might write a general overview of your subject, or choose to focus down on a specific part of it. You may be asked specifically to write on a subject or an aspect of your subject by a publisher or editor. Whatever you write is **your** take, **your** perspective and **your** bias on the subject chosen. Even if you think that what you write is uncontentious and accepted by the majority, you have to be prepared to defend your position, backing up your argument in a non-fiction book just as you would in an article for a journal. Check all your facts again and ensure that your advice is current and accurate.

Be prepared for criticism from people who hold different opinions to yourself, as in Box 2.1. You will have to develop a tough hide as a writer in order to tolerate critical reviews which may display the ignorance of the reviewer or the fact that they had merely scanned the book, while at the same time you need to listen and respond to well thought out feedback.

Box 2.1

Having striven to write a simple easy book on a complex subject, it is galling to receive a criticism:

'The presentation is repetitive and somewhat superficial. This comment may be harsh but perhaps a small book such as this cannot be expected to be both simple and erudite.'

As a novice

If you have only a basic grasp of a subject, then you could write a book as you explore the field. Your perspective will be a new one. You will spot difficulties that readers will come across as they are learning about a topic, whereas an expert may have forgotten the problems and issues that loom large to someone just starting out. You should be able to write in a readable manner. You will not be bogged down with jargon, as you will not have been in the field long enough to be using it unconsciously – and you will know not to blind other novices like yourself with important-sounding words that are unfamiliar to you and that neither you nor your readers understand.

Some writers who are novices in the field write their book as a diary – recording their pathway to experience. It might be about solving a problem or carrying out a project with some key goals.

Get on with putting the book proposal together and starting writing while you are driven to do so. It is tempting to procrastinate until an arbitrary time, such as the end of a job, project or your career, when you think you will have more time. However, it does not work out that way. Other things will crop up, like a new project or idea, or you will have less energy for driving your writing due to time pressures at work. Your creative ideas may dry up if they are not part of the buzz of a busy working life.

A one-off book or can you run to a series?

You may begin by writing a book as one stand-alone 'project'. But once you have embarked on the book, you might find that there is too much material for one book. In that case you could split the contents into two parallel books, as Ruth and Gill did in Box 2.2.

Box 2.2

Ruth and Gill were writing a book about clinical governance. But in describing the learning culture needed to establish clinical governance, they generated a great many ideas and much material about education and training. So they split the contents into a book on continuing professional development[1] and another on clinical governance,[2] with about ten per cent of each book containing similar material.

So you may evolve a cluster of books in this way, or you could set out with a plan for a series of books with the same purpose and intended readership but on varied subjects – as Ruth and Gill did in Box 2.3.

Box 2.3

Ruth and Gill set out to write a series of books to meet doctors' requirements for their forthcoming revalidation, by guiding them in how they could demonstrate their competence and good performance in more than 30 clinical fields.[3] They planned these books for GPs in the first instance, but then extended the series by involving co-authors. Two consultants in reproductive health joined them to produce a book to help consultants and specialist registrars demonstrate their competence, and two primary care nurses helped to revise the material in the GP series for nurses, extending the series by another four books. Extending the series was not part of the original plan, but the GP books were so good and useful that the opportunity was taken to convert them for nurse and hospital doctor readerships, too.

Writing for the general reader

Writing a book based on a project or a thesis usually implies that you are writing for a specialist reader – one who will pick up your book because the title has words in it that already interest the reader, as in Box 2.4.

Box 2.4 Titles of interest to a specialist reader

Clinical Audit in Primary Care[4]
Someone who is interested in, or knows they have to do, clinical audit and who works in primary care.

Improving Sexual Health Advice[5]
Someone who is interested in sexual health and who needs to know how to advise people about it.

A Compendium of Health Statistics[6]
This title is likely to appeal to a narrower range of readers – for libraries, and researchers into healthcare trends.

Some titles need explanations to direct them to a specialist or general reader.

Box 2.5

The cover of *How Drugs Work*[7] has to tell the reader that it is directed at 'those who have prescribing responsibilities, such as nurse prescribers, general practitioners, pharmacists and dentists; nurses who require an understanding of drug actions and interactions; and pharmaceutical industry representatives.'

The title *How Drugs Work* (*see* Box 2.5) could equally well have been directed towards the lay person in the general community, but would have required a very different content and style.

Academics who want to write for a wider general audience can easily see the advantages. If this is done well, the book will have more readers, sell more copies, generate more publicity and attention, and more royalties. The downside is less obvious. Academic institutions and fellow academics are not kind to 'popular' writers if they have become successful and well known. This is less of a problem if the author has already produced several 'academic' books. Perhaps the rest of the academics believe that the general reader is less critical and more likely to accept poor argument or evidence for ideas. It is as though, by writing well for a general audience, you have devalued your specialist knowledge. If you are unsuccessful in writing a book for the general reader, this is not surprising. It is extremely difficult for someone who is a real expert on their subject to write simply enough for non-specialists to understand them.

If you want to try this route, spend some time reading books written for the general reader. Absorb the style, the straightforward language and, above all, the simplicity of the argument that you are proposing. It is likely that you will find that a book for the general reader (*see* Box 2.6) makes only a few points but explains and illustrates them in many different ways.

Box 2.6

Beat Back Pain (52 Brilliant Ideas)[8] contains many different and interesting ways of saying 'exercise improves back pain.'

You will also find that book reviewers are pitiless towards academic writers of general non-fiction. Even the smallest injection of theoretical language, specialised language or, worse still, statistics or a formula, will incur great vilification. Any book that requires a glossary to explain the terms or language used will have a restricted readership.

Writing humorously for the general reader is also fraught with pitfalls. Even if you have written amusing short pieces for a lightweight healthcare magazine, you will find that it is much more difficult to write a whole book in a light-hearted way without causing offence. What passes for humour among your own colleagues may well be regarded as offensive to other people, as can be clearly seen from correspondence following the publication of satirical pieces in journals.

Writing for the specialist reader

First, define your reader. Although you will never be published if you do not please the publisher, you will never write a good book, or even a reasonable one, unless you know your target audience. Just as you need to consider how to write for the general reader, your content and style must be directed at those whom you want to read what you write. The wider you want your readership to be, the simpler your language must be. If you want to put someone off, write turgid text laced with technical terms (*see* Box 2.7).

Box 2.7

Put your readers off with:
Using a pluralistic methodology the findings provide a combination of the

---

subjective and objective views intermittently within the research cycles, thereby giving the researcher a more holistic view of this research.

Instead of:
Using both subjective and objective methods helps the researcher to have a more rounded view.

If you target your audience poorly, you will invite criticisms such as that in Box 2.8.

Box 2.8

'*The Vaccine Controversy* often lacks essential detail in important areas and contains too little referenced material for a professional audience. Nor does it have the parents' point of view you might expect for a lay readership.'[9]

What type of book?

Consider carefully what type of book you want to write. Go and look at the relevant shelves in a bookshop for ideas. Look at the categories in an online bookstore or in a publisher's catalogue. It could be:

- an expression of a point of view or a philosophical argument (e.g. *Rationing Medical Care on the Basis of Age*[10])
- a book based on your thesis (e.g. *Sexual Health Matters in Primary Care*[11])
- a general textbook (e.g. *Oxford Textbook of Primary Medical Care*[12])
- a specialist textbook (e.g. *Infant Feeding and Nutrition for Primary Care*[13])
- a 'toolkit' text (e.g. *Coaching for Effective Learning*[14])
- a synopsis or brief notes on a subject (e.g. *Medicine at a Glance*[15])
- a reference resource (e.g. *A Compendium of Health Statistics*[6])
- a narrative account (e.g. *Life After Darkness*[16])
- a historical book (e.g. *John MacAlister's Other Vision*[17]).

Define your **purpose**, **audience** and **format** for each. Do not confuse and irritate the reader by combining different types of book. A narrative account and a historical book combine well, but beware of trying to combine a toolkit and a textbook, or an opinion-based book and a textbook. You will provoke an adverse reaction!

An expression of a point of view or a philosophical argument

You may be part of a committee examining ethical dilemmas, or have written a thesis on an ethical theme. You may have become incensed by lack of equity or opportunity in health availability or in jobs. You will need to know your subject well and have spent time debating it with others. Your book is likely to be topical, it may have arisen out of media headlines, and it will need to be written quickly on the basis of already completed investigation and research.

Converting your expert knowledge in a thesis to a book

You may, like many authors, start by writing a book on the subject of your thesis. You are already an expert by virtue of having done the research and defended your thesis against criticism. Do not make the mistake of arguing your case again. The literature search has to go. Your defensive arguments must be turned to positive, persuasive statements. Your references must be easily accessible to the reader, not used to demonstrate that your search for evidence has reached the most obscure journals. Dissertations have long lists of citations, far more than anyone other than your examiners would wish to read. They may demonstrate your research skills – but a reference is only necessary if the point you propose makes the reader think 'How does he/she know that? What is the evidence for that statement?'. If you are not laying out the evidence yourself in the text, then you need to provide the reference on which it is based.

Your thesis was couched in negative terms, seeking to disprove a hypothesis – the negative framing of the important research question. Now you must put the question and its answer at the outset of the book, to capture the reader's attention right at the beginning. The rest of the book provides the detail explaining why you have come to believe that your answer is correct.

Box 2.9 Changing the emphasis from thesis to book

The title of a thesis called

> *'The quality of life in the community for patients previously in a long-stay psychiatric hospital'*

had as its hypothesis

> *'The quality of life in the community for patients compared with when they were previously in a long-stay psychiatric hospital would not show any improvement.'*

For a book title, you would need to change this argument into

> *'Life in the community is better for patients who were previously in long-stay hospital care'*

(so long as that reflects what the thesis showed!).

Using large sections of previous researchers' work to illustrate agreement or otherwise with the argument in your thesis is common. In a book, you should keep quotations from other people's work to a minimum and show them clearly for what they are – not your work. Use quotation marks and reference the source. Plagiarism is using another's work without crediting it to them, and is unethical. Plagiarism is stealing someone's work and passing it off as your own. If you paraphrase, you must still give the reference, as you are not referring to your work but to that of another author.

Many dissertations consist of an introduction and then several applications (projects or arguments) to attempt to demonstrate the answer. This format frequently has no obvious conclusion apart from 'more research is needed.' The conclusion is full of new questions that the research or exploration of the original premise revealed. A definite answer to the question first posed is frequently not obtained, but this is acceptable because the thesis is about the journey of discovery to the answer that there is no definite answer. A book based on such a thesis needs much reworking. If you are considering writing a book based on this type of thesis, try writing the first chapter, where you lay out your question, and the last chapter, where you summarise the answer. You must have a much greater capacity for fine and fluid writing if you hope to hold your reader to an inconclusive ending without incurring disappointment, especially if your thesis is long and often couched in 'academic' language. Spend time teasing out the main exciting point that started you off on the research – this excitement is what you need to transmit to your reader. Write about that. If you have no enthusiasm left for the subject, you will write a boring book, so stop now and think what else you could write. You will need to rewrite what you have already written in the thesis because you have a different audience. Keep in mind the **purpose** – to transfer some of what you found out about this exciting question to others – and your **audience** – decide whether the 'others' are in your specialist field or if you are writing for the more general reader. Then you can think about the **format** – how you will organise the book and the style you want to use.

A general or specialist textbook

Look at your competitors. What can you add that is unique? Can you have a distinct **purpose** that is different from that of other textbooks? Can you slant it towards an **audience** that has not been considered by other writers? What about having a **format** that leaps out as user-friendly (*see* Box 2.10)?

Box 2.10

What not to do:

> An author persuaded a publisher to issue an atlas of all his collection of slides of breast lesions. It was neither a coffee-table book nor a reference book, and with no text to guide the reader, it was repetitive and unselected. It was not a success.

What to do:

> Put your chapters on a searchable CD or a palmtop programme issued with the book to give added value and help people to use it more easily.

Consider collaborating with at least one other person in your field. Writing a textbook on your own can lead you to omit important facets of the subject. You may prefer to be an editor and ask others to write on their particular areas of interest, but look at Chapter 3 to find out about the pitfalls of this approach. Recognise that the book will be out of date the day you finish doing the research for it, and build in time and space to add revisions as new material is published in journals.

A toolkit of your project

If your book relates to a project, is it about you capturing what you have learned to help others to avoid your mistakes, or to disseminate the practical materials you have put together for others to use? Do you wait until you have finished the project or do you write it up as you go along?

The answer probably depends on how organised you are. The more notes you take as you go along, the better you will capture the dilemmas that occurred as you progressed, and how you overcame any obstacles. By the end of the project, you may have a rosy view of the project's progress throughout and have forgotten your thoughts and doubts along the way, unless you have a contemporaneous record of them. You could be writing up chapters of the book in draft, ready to revise it quite harshly as you complete the manuscript. If you are writing the book as the project progresses, it will be difficult to judge how many words to spend on the first stages of your project or to get a balance between the initial, middle and final stages of the project, when you are not yet aware how things will work out.

Your enthusiasm and excitement about being part of a burgeoning project will show through in your writing if you are completing the manuscript as you go along, rather than reflecting back from the safety of its completion.

The thrust of your project might be the evidence you produced of how to make changes happen. In that case, you will have to leave most of the writing until you have finished the project and know it is worth writing about. The majority of the book will be streamlined to focus on how to undertake the planning and tasks that led to the changes, and it will be easier to complete the book proposal and manuscript with the benefit of hindsight about what worked.

A synopsis or brief notes

These brief outlines may seem superficially attractive to the expert. You think that you will not have to write much and, after all, you know your subject inside out. But if you are an expert, this is one of the most difficult types of book to write. By the time you are an expert, you know all the 'exceptions to the rule.' You want to say 'generally this applies, but occasionally you will find . . .'. There is no room for this in a synopsis of the subject!

The time to write a synopsis or outline might be when you are competent in the subject, but not yet aware of all the occasions on which the information or guidelines fail to cover the situation. Such a book is often best written by someone who knows what they need to learn about a new subject, researches it, and then writes what they found was important to know. Be prepared for criticism from experts, who will always find exceptions to the necessarily dogmatic statements in a synopsis. The experts who criticise the synopsis or brief notes will also think that you should have included a lot more because, as you become more expert, you forget what is core to beginners.

A reference work

This is the only place for all those statistics or tables that you have laboriously collected. It must be meticulously researched and checked again and again. Make sure that it has a **purpose** for **others** before embarking on such a momentous task. It is expensive to produce and has a limited **audience** and a boring **format**. It is a minority market and likely to be your only publication.

A narrative account

This is a biography or autobiography with a message. A biography allows you to use detailed research into a case history, or perhaps several, to illustrate what an illness or disability is like from the perspective of the sufferer or carer. You may have a story of your own to tell about suffering from an illness, or caring for someone with one, and the triumphs and vicissitudes encountered along the way. Consider your **purpose**. If it is vindictive, you risk losing the reader's sympathy. Are your solutions or proposals right for other people as well? What you are proposing to change must be practicable.

What about your **audience**? You might want to target other people with similar complaints, people who work in the health service or those who decide or implement government policy. Think carefully about the **format**. If you write in the first person, the writing is immediate, often heart-rending, but sometimes dismissed as over-emotional if your targets are administrators or professionals. Writing in the third person can sound odd if it is a personal account, but is more acceptable for a biography or a collection of case histories. Third-person writing distances you from the subject matter and the emotion a little, so is less powerful, but can help to make a rational argument or proposal more acceptable.

A historical book

If you have an interest in how things began, how they developed, or a connection with a particular event, person, building or institution, this is an ideal topic. You must be accurate, so do your research. Establish whether you have enough material for a book – if the subject matter is brief, change your ideas into an article. Your **purpose** is clear – to tell the general reader about an event that happened or a person who lived in the past and influenced the present. If it has no contempory resonance or relevance, focus on the interest and excitement of the discovery. Define your **audience** carefully. The subject may be of general interest or appeal to only a narrow cross-section of general readers. The **format** will be more like an extended essay or a detective story than a textbook. Avoid technical language and extend your potential readership.

Writing a chapter for someone else's book

If someone approaches you to invite you to write one or more chapters for their book, and you are already an established writer, what is in it for you? Do you really want four free books from the publisher's list or a £100 cheque in two years' time? These incentives are not enough. So look at your other reasons for agreeing to write:

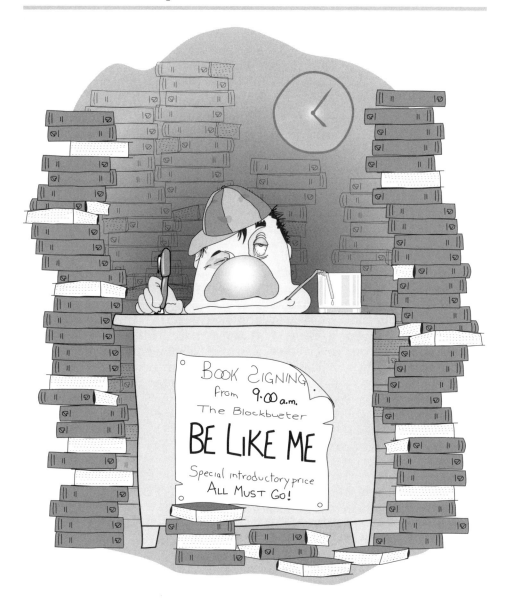

- you have important points to make and this book will give you the opportunity to express them
- you feel obliged to the person asking you because they have done you favours in the past
- you have a sense of duty to the readership
- you think that you will do it better than anyone else who might be asked.

If you are not an established writer, this may give you an opportunity to dip your toe in the water. The above reasons may also apply. Recognise that an edited book may take at least two years to be published. You could be writing your own book in that time.

References

1 Wakley G, Chambers R. *Continuing Professional Development in Primary Care*. Oxford: Radcliffe Medical Press; 2000.
2 Chambers R, Wakley G. *Making Clinical Governance Work for You*. Oxford: Radcliffe Medical Press; 2000.
3 Wakley G, Chambers R and various co-authors. *Demonstrating Your Competence* series. Oxford: Radcliffe Publishing; 2004–2006.
4 Chambers R, Wakley G. *Clinical Audit in Primary Care*. Oxford: Radcliffe Publishing; 2005.
5 Wakley G, Cunnion M, Chambers R. *Improving Sexual Health Advice*. Oxford: Radcliffe Medical Press; 2003.
6 Yuen P. *A Compendium of Health Statistics*. Oxford: Radcliffe Publishing; 2005.
7 McGavock H. *How Drugs Work*. Oxford: Radcliffe Publishing; 2005.
8 Chambers R. *Beat Back Pain (52 Brilliant Ideas)*. Oxford: Infinite Ideas Ltd; 2004.
9 Roberts R. Book review of Link K. *The Vaccine Controversy*. Praeger. *BMJ*. 2005; **331**: 1209.
10 Matthews E, Russell E. *Rationing Medical Care on the Basis of Age*. Oxford: Radcliffe Publishing; 2005.
11 Wakley G, Chambers R. *Sexual Health Matters in Primary Care*. Oxford: Radcliffe Medical Press; 2002.
12 Jones R, Britten N, Culpepper L *et al.* (eds) *Oxford Textbook of Primary Medical Care*. Oxford: Oxford University Press; 2005.
13 Bentley D, Aubrey S, Bentley M. *Infant Feeding and Nutrition for Primary Care*. Oxford: Radcliffe Publishing; 2004.
14 Claridge M, Lewis T. *Coaching for Effective Learning*. Oxford: Radcliffe Publishing; 2005.
15 Davey P. *Medicine at a Glance*. 2nd ed. Oxford: Blackwell Publishing; 2003.
16 Wield C. *Life After Darkness: a doctor's journey through severe depression*. Oxford: Radcliffe Publishing; 2006.
17 Cook GC. *John MacAlister's Other Vision*. Oxford: Radcliffe Publishing; 2006.

Chapter 3

In what capacity will you be writing?

Ruth Chambers

Selecting your role

You could have a major or minor role in writing the book. You might be the editor or one of the co-editors, the sole author, one of two or more co-authors, a chapter contributor of a part of one or more chapters, or you may be simply writing the foreword for the book.

If you are leading the book 'project' then you will be choosing the role that suits you – that matches your interest or expertise, your preference, your skills in writing or project management, your capacity to accommodate the work and your own or others' timescales. Which role you take on will also depend on *why* you are writing the book – matched to the types of reasons for writing a book that were described in Chapters 1 and 2. Your role will depend on whether it is a 'project' initiated by you, whether it is expected of you, or the nature of the person or organisation that has asked you to take on the writing. If you are writing it to enhance your academic or expert status, for example, then you are going to want to be one of the main authors or the editor of the book.

The reason we are referring to the writing of the book as a 'project' will become clearer as you take in all the information in this book. You will realise that all the various facets involved must be well coordinated for a successful and timely product – your published book – whether you are a main author or an editor.

Another factor to take into account when selecting your role in writing the book is your personality. Many authors are by nature introverts, according to the description within the Myers–Briggs personality profile.[1] This means that their heads are packed with ideas and developments, in contrast to the extrovert personality, whose ideas are very much drawn from others and their external environment. An introvert might strongly prefer to write their own material. An extrovert might be happy to edit the work written by others, drawing from their ideas or in addition to writing their own text. Knowing your Myers–Briggs personality profile will give you other leads about the kinds of writing you are comfortable with. For instance, those with a strong personality bias towards 'feeling' might be comfortable specialising in narratives, or those with a personality profile tending towards 'judging' might opt for an academic approach to writing that demands evidence to underpin their texts.

Being an editor: some insights

To be a successful editor you need to be a well-organised person. You should be good at giving constructive and timely feedback, with plenty of patience for chivvying your writers along to complete sections of work that they have contracted to do for you. You will have to be flexible and able to renegotiate what a particular chapter author can manage if their circumstances change or they can no longer fulfil what was agreed. You need to be firm without being bossy, and give a critical review of their work based on facts rather than on your subjective feelings.

If you are the sort of person who does not rate their organisational or people management skills very highly, then you would be best avoiding the editing role. It involves much chasing of successive draft chapters from scatterbrained people like you who are the contributors.

If you are highly introverted, you might find it difficult to act as editor if you believe that you could have written the chapters that contributors submit to you in different or 'better' ways. You might not be able to sit back and let various contributors lead on the content of their chapters without insisting on major changes or shifts of emphasis, or rewriting the whole lot. You must value their work and demonstrate this. The reason you are editing the book instead of writing it first hand is that the book will be richer and more useful for readers if it has the diverse experience and input of the various contributors.

If you are an introvert, you may have too few contacts and networks in any case to be able to pull a book proposal together where you are the editor for a range of experienced and eminent writers. You may need to 'get out more' first at conferences, working groups, or other academic or health and social care environments before you can expect to assume the role of editor. Even if such conferences or meetings scare you or bore you, force yourself to build up networks of people with mutual interests or expertise that complement your own.

Those authors who are contributing chapters will have to know you and trust you with their work – and as writing a chapter or two is often additional to someone's day job, the editor needs to inspire commitment. Your chapter authors will need to respect your judgement and have confidence in your ability as an editor or co-editor. After all, they will be submitting their work to your 'red pen.' You will have the final say in the edited material – especially what you decide should be left out. They will have the last word on any concepts or position statements in their chapter(s), as the material will be attributed to their name, but how those concepts and statements are relayed will be agreed between the writer and the editor. You will either need to have reasonable expertise in the topics they are writing about, or know someone who does who is prepared to peer review an individual chapter, to be able to act as a 'critical friend' to your writers so that they respect your judgement about content and emphasis. You may be able to buddy up one contributor with another, to review each other's work, if you do not have sufficient background to critique it. You will then be the one to decide, if the contributor who is reviewing disagrees with the writer and they cannot agree on a middle ground.

You need to stay up to date in the field while the book is being written by your contributory authors, so that you can spot a gap or out-of-date material as best you can. You should understand, too, any biases that your authors have and be able to judge whether you need to suggest additions or revisions to rectify this. Table 3.1 is an example of such bias written by someone who prefers being a main author to editing a book. The sole authorship emphasises the buzz she gets from

Table 3.1 A view of the pros and cons of editing or being a main author of a book

Main author	Editor
Pros	
1 You can develop and shape the text as you want it	1 You can sit back (to some extent) while other people write the book
2 It is your text so you experience the excitement and buzz from your creativity and reflections that generate new ideas	2 Other writers have diverse experience and opinions and provide a breadth of material and expertise that extends the scope of the book
3 You can dictate the speed of writing and progress through the different stages in preparing for and undertaking the writing and proof checking of the book	3 You have the opportunity to enjoy and savour other people's writing on subjects in which you are interested as you work through editing the contributed chapters in minute detail
4 You are accountable for your own work – no one to blame but yourself if you get something wrong	
Cons	
1 You may have underestimated the time and effort involved in undertaking solo or co-authored writing of the book. You could end up giving up halfway through and wasting your effort	1 You are dependent on others fulfilling their pledges to send you chapters or sections with the agreed content and to time
2 If you are writing alone, you have no one to intimately peer review the manuscript and warn you about gaps or mistakes or false claims	2 Editing may take far longer than you budgeted for, especially if contributory authors are slow or send successive drafts for your feedback or produce incomplete or scanty work
	3 If you are not an expert on the topic a contributing author is writing on, you are dependent on them for accurate and reliable text, or on finding peer reviewers who are prepared to give their time freely
	4 Editing requires intense organisation for which you might have insufficient skills and patience

writing herself. Someone who enjoys editing derives quiet satisfaction from pulling together other people's work into a coordinated whole.

Your life as an editor will be easier if you set out from the start a realistic timetable and your requirements about the scope and depth of each chapter. Share this information about all of the chapters with each contributor in order to minimise duplication, so that they can see whether some of what they intend to write about is being covered in another chapter. If they persist in wanting to write about a topic that is outside the scope of their chapter, negotiate between authors to redefine their respective chapters. Define the purpose of the book and the audience. The nature of the expected readership should be made clear, so that all contributors are writing for the same audience and know at what level of prior knowledge and understanding to pitch their writing.

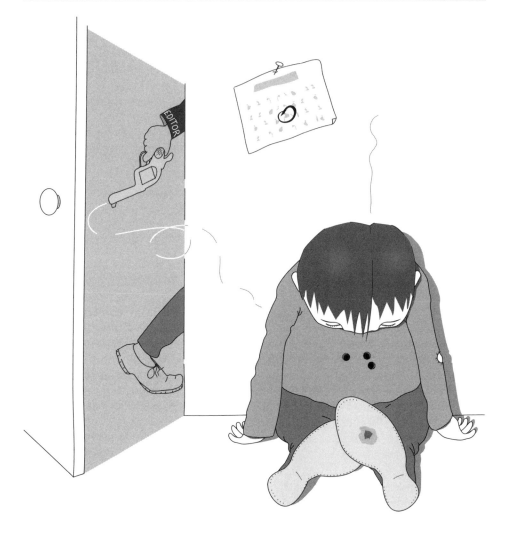

He never met his deadlines.

Describe the format and style you want, too. Perhaps it is to be an easy-read type of style with short sentences and popular words, using 'you' when advising the reader. If it is an academic treatise, the writing should still flow easily but be more objective, and statements and ideas should be referenced. If there are to be references, explain the publisher's style (*see* Box 3.1) and give some examples of how to prepare the references for an article, a book, an unpublished report and a personal anecdote. Find out as much as you can about the publisher's in-house style and share that information with your authors. Entreat them to read and adhere to the style guidance even if it differs from their usual practice.

Box 3.1

Radcliffe Publishing have now adopted the Vancouver style of referencing[2] to replace their previous in-house style. This makes it much easier for authors who store and sort the references to publications in their fields of interest using electronic software such as Reference Manager, Endnote or RefViz, as they can simply copy appropriate references into their writing.

Let your chapter contributor know whether the format is suitable for them to write as if giving personal experience and guidance using an 'I did this . . .' style of text. Be firm about the need to include case studies or examples of 'how to do it' to break up the text. Let your authors know about any rules on the use of jargon and abbreviations, so that everyone is using the same approach. All this will minimise the amount of editing and revision you have to do and will make your life easier so long as your authors stick to your requirements.

Table 3.1 describes some of the key differences between being the editor and a main author of a book. Of course, it is not an either/or choice. You may write one or more chapters of a book you are editing, especially if one of the contributors lets you down and you cannot find a substitute author at short notice, or you are the expert on one of the fields that the book covers.

Time and planning issues of editing jump out of Table 3.1. So it is best to make a timetabled plan for your editing role, as in the Gantt chart shown in Figure 3.1. The various key tasks of being an editor and the way you interact with the authors and publisher are listed here, with possible time spans against each task. Different publishers take longer or shorter times to complete their part in the publication process. For example, the agreeing and issuing of the book proposal in Figure 3.1 is shown as happening over a two-week period, whereas some publishers may take three to six months to peer review the book proposal and gauge marketing opportunities before commissioning a book. Even erring on the side of estimating minimal times, the time span for editing a book from the time of the concept of the book to its publication is nearly two years in this example.

You will see that an editor's tasks include helping the publisher with the promotion of the published book. This responsibility is likely to include compiling the book promotion questionnaire for the publisher so that they can publicise the forthcoming book at book fairs and in their advertising material, thereby maximising its profile and opportunities for bulk sales or retail outlets selling the book. Later you might help to seek organisations or publications likely to

Tasks (for editor unless specified)	April	July	Oct	Jan	April	July	Oct	Jan
• Draft book proposal, invite authors and agree input, submit to publisher.	→→→→→→→							
• Publisher issues contracts for agreed book proposal.			→					
• Set out agreed requirements for authors: style, scope, timing, etc.			→					
• Contributory authors write chapters/submit to editor.			→→→→→→→					
• Complete book promotion questionnaire for publisher, involving authors.			→→					
• Chivvy writers who are late submitting.					→→→→			
• Maintain contact with contributory writers, communicating progress.			→→→→→→→→→→→→→→→					
• Edit chapters as received, referring back to authors for revisions, references, additions; checking final product.				→→→→				
• Submit final manuscript after intense editing of whole.						→		
• Respond to editor/author queries by publisher.						→→		
• Check copy-edited proof of manuscript.							→	
• Publish book.								→
• Write profile-raising articles, give interviews, hold related workshops, etc.							→→→→	

Two year period: by quarters

Figure 3.1 Example of timetabled project plan for editing a book.

nominate someone to review the book and publish a piece about it. Writing articles linked to the book can also be a great way to increase awareness, and therefore sales, of the book.

Being a main author or co-author: some insights

Think whether you love both writing itself and the topic of your projected book enough to devote the estimated minimum of 24 x 10-hour days of time gauged for an experienced solo author of a 50,000-word book, as described in Box 1.1. If you doubt your commitment or capacity, then why not co-author with one or more other authors whose writing you trust and respect? Or if it is just a capacity issue, then maybe you could find regular writing time over a longer period, such as a year, instead of the shorter timescales shown in Figure 3.2. Of course, then you might be risking the initial material becoming out of date and burdening you with considerable updating, or other authors and publishers producing a similar book that hits the market first.

Table 3.2 captures some of the pros and cons of being a solo author or writing jointly with others. Four is probably the maximum number of authors for a book, where you all jointly own it. It is more usual to have two or three co-authors. One of you will have to act as the lead with regard to managing the book-writing process, relating to the publisher, and probably being the one to edit the manuscript as a whole.

Co-authors need to act as a team, with everyone knowing what their role and responsibilities are and how they fit with the others. It will be important for you all to get on with each other and respect each others' views and writing. There would be no point in co-authors with conflicting views writing together unless that was the essence of the book – presenting two or more perspectives of a situation. Otherwise there would be likely to be intense argument throughout the book-writing process, conducted in a counter-productive manner.

If you are a set of co-authors, make your action plan together, agreeing who does what for the key tasks such as those included in the Gantt chart in Figure 3.2, with corresponding time deadlines and milestones. If one author lets the other(s) down by, for instance, not completing the promised chapters or input, then the team leader will have to be decisive about how to react. The reason for non-completion will be pertinent to the action that you take. For example, if a co-author's computer has been faulty, or their close relative has died or they are in the midst of a messy divorce, you and they should have a good idea of how long the delay in submitting their share of the writing will be. If it is likely to be only a short delay, you will probably choose to postpone the completion of the book manuscript for a similarly short period. If it will be a protracted delay or perhaps they will be unable to complete the writing, you have other options. You can find a replacement writer, one of the other co-authors could take it on, or you could reshape the contents of the book, with the publisher's agreement, and omit or replace the subjects about which your absentee co-author was going to write.

If you are a solo author, you should still compose an action plan with milestones and deadlines to help you plan and monitor your progress. This should enable you to keep abreast of the writing and other tasks that you need to do in order to meet the publisher's deadlines. You could determine whether you have any learning needs yourself, in writing the book. Then integrate any learning activities you plan to do in your Gantt chart – perhaps meeting up for a discussion with an experienced author, attending an advanced 'how to publish' course or attending a course on other aspects of writing expertise.

Some of the pros and cons of choosing to be a solo author or having co-authors are presented in Table 3.2.

Authors need to enjoy the writing and revel in the opportunity to be creative and construct their own work. They should enjoy the opportunity to broadcast their own views and experiences, and to value the written word as a method of communication instead of or as well as the spoken word (as in speeches or more visual communication).

Table 3.2 Some pros and cons of solo writing or co-authoring a book

Solo writing	*Co-authored writing*
Pros	
1 You are in charge of the scope, emphases, opinions, etc. expressed in the book	1 It is fun and comradely to have one or more co-authors with whom you are in a writing team, providing support and ideas for each other
2 You are in charge of the timetable of writing – and can plan your life around it and write at your own pace	2 Other writers have diverse experience and opinions and provide a breadth of material and expertise that extends the scope of the book beyond what you can write on your own
3 If anything goes wrong with the writing process, you can make unanimous decisions about what action to take!	3 You can add your other ideas to other people's chapters and you'll enjoy their comments and suggestions that enrich your work, too
4 You can keep all the royalties yourself – there are no other authors to share these funds with	4 Your joint networks are more than your solo network in terms of identifying marketing opportunities, recruiting someone to write the foreword, finding avenues for peer reviews of the book, and running linked workshops
5 You are the one communicating with the publisher about the publication process or marketing – so there is less chance of miscommunication	5 You have teammates to help you push yourself to meet writing deadlines so that you don't let others down
6 It is *your* project, and that feels good	
7 There is no need to worry whether any other writer agrees with your style, approach or perspective	
Cons	
1 Being a solo author is a lonely business, and you might give up writing the book halfway through without others to urge and cajole you	1 You might fall out as co-authors over some minor or major matter that disrupts the writing process or stops it altogether
2 There is no one to take a real constructive interest in what you are writing and to challenge weak areas or spot mistakes	2 One or more co-authors may fail to agree over a principle or concept that makes the book unworkable, with alternative models being advocated in different chapters in illogical ways
3 A great deal of work is involved in writing a book alone, and if you lose your excitement and creativity under the workload you might end up with a dull book	3 Co-authors may have such different styles that the book lacks coherence despite editing
	4 One co-author may not recognise a team writer as the lead with the final say on editing the manuscript
	5 The writing team leader may have poor people-handling skills, so that their leadership and overall editing are undertaken without regard to co-authors' views and feelings

Two year period: by quarters

Tasks (for authors unless specified)	April	July	Oct	Jan	April	July	Oct	Jan
• Draft book proposal, agree author's input, who will edit, submit to publisher.	•———		→→					
• Publisher issues contracts for agreed book proposal.			→					
• Authors agree: style, scope, timing, etc.			→					
• Joint authors write chapters/ swop and review each others' work, agreeing revisions, additions.			•———	→				
• Complete book promotion questionnaire for publisher, involving authors.			→					
• Submit final manuscript after intense editing of whole as joint or lead task.					→			
• Respond to editor/author queries by publisher.					•———	→		
• Check copy-edited proof of manuscript.						→		
• Publish book.							→	
• Write profile-raising articles, give interviews, hold related workshops, etc.							•———	→

Figure 3.2 Example of timetabled project plan for being joint author of a book.

Figure 3.2 gives examples of time periods for each stage of writing a book as a joint author. Writing as a joint author is represented here as taking several months' less time than editing a book with a variety of contributing authors (as shown in Figure 3.1).

So have a go. There are pros and cons to being the editor, the solo author or one of two or more co-authors. Some of these will depend on your circumstances, some on your expertise and that which is needed, and some on your preferences and your own style. Why not give them all a go, as once you have written a book you will probably be hooked and want to start again – this time learning from last time and not falling into the same traps or making the same mistakes (or so you think!)?

Time to complete your writing

In reality, the time component for any writing will depend on how quickly you can write drafts and edit your completed manuscript. Your circumstances will vary at different stages of your life – and with your commitments at home and work. If you are an academic with a post in a higher education institution, you might have protected work time for writing. If you are a teacher, you might have gaps between courses for preparation when you can incorporate some time spent

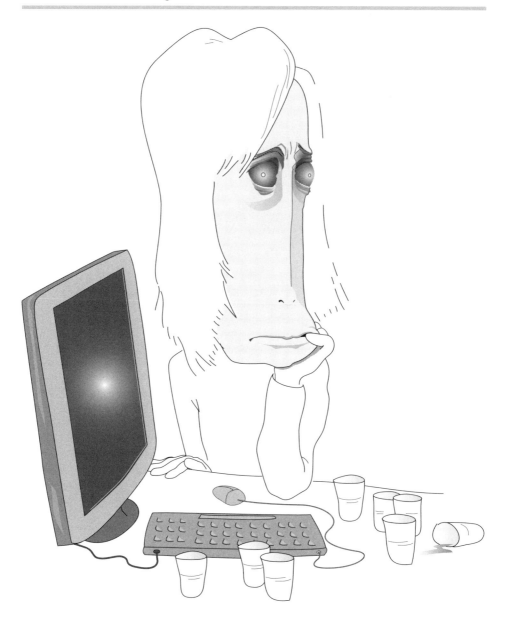

The trouble with reflection is that I keep thinking that I could
be doing something more interesting.

writing your book. If you are working more than full-time already you might be relying on days of annual leave or weekends and evenings for time and space to do all your writing. Another factor that determines how long it will take you is the extent to which you will be carrying out research while you are writing – for evidence, case studies, examples of people's experiences, etc.

Reflection takes time, too. You might not be able to rush from writing one chapter to the next. You may need time to brood about the topic you are writing on next, to consider your approach, and to think out your take on it and how you will structure your writing. Then you will need to reflect on successive drafts to improve and extend the chapter, before you consider it completed and can advance to the next one. Alternatively, you may be able to work better by writing more than one chapter in parallel, feeding from one into another. Another factor that influences the time taken for writing is the degree to which what you are writing about is original, or how much it is based on collating and adapting other people's materials or published texts. An able personal assistant who can assist with the research for evidence or case studies, or type up some of your jottings or handwritten diagrams, can also speed the writing along.

References

1 Myers IB, Myers P. *Gifts Differing. Understanding personality type*. Palo Alto, California: Davies-Black Publishing; 1980.
2 Radcliffe Publishing Ltd. *Guide for Authors*. Oxford: Radcliffe Publishing; 2006. www. radcliffe-oxford.com

Chapter 4

How to write a convincing book proposal

Ruth Chambers

What is it for?

If this is your first time, ask others who have put a book proposal together to share with you the template and approach that they use. They will undoubtedly have links to various publishers and have developed their usual book-proposal template to match a particular publisher's in-house requirements, or proposal form, as in Box 4.3 at the end of this chapter.

The aim of your book proposal is to sell the main ideas and scope of your book. Make the publisher you are approaching feel confident that there will be a good market for the book you are offering. Very occasionally, publishers do commission a book as a 'loss leader' knowing that potential sales are limited because the likely readership is small. This is rare, and will only be for personal reasons such as completing the publisher's repertoire of books, or because the publisher is committed to the particular field of the book, perhaps for altruistic or charitable reasons.

Do some intense market research

Your market research will help you to justify the extent of time and effort you and any other authors will put into researching and writing the book, as well as collating the justification for your book proposal. This market research will include searching publisher databases and their catalogues, and hunting through websites of book sales companies to identify and critique any books that might be competitive or complementary to the one you propose. Chat to a variety of people who could be your future readers so that you can shape the scope and contents of the book to meet their needs. Check out their perspectives on your planned book. Ask them about the changes they expect from forthcoming legislation, or national or local policies, which could herald reorganisations and new ways of working that in turn create a new niche for your proposed book.

How to convince a publisher to accept your book proposal

You need to do several tasks in parallel.

1 Find the right publisher to approach about your proposed book
2 Identify appropriate authors to write with you

3 Prepare your book proposal in the way that a particular publisher expects or requires

You are looking for a particular publisher who is right for your field and your readership and has a space for your book. Some of the information that you need will come from networking with other authors and publishers, a key component of your intense market research. Some help might come from publications such as the *Writers' and Artists' Yearbook*,[1] which is a directory for writers and others that lists publishers in the UK and elsewhere and describes their market, giving the names and contact details of managing and editorial staff (*see* Box 4.1 for an example which shows the entry for Radcliffe Publishing).

If you have a literary agent (*see* Chapter 6) or maybe a mentor who is giving you the benefit of their experience, they could help you to redraft and reshape your book proposal to one that is likely to be snapped up by the publisher(s) to whom you submit it.

Box 4.1 Entry for Radcliffe Publishing in the *Writers' and Artists' Yearbook*[1]

18 Marcham Road, Abingdon, Oxon OX14 1AA
tel (01235) 528820 *fax* (01235) 528830
email contact.us@radcliffemed.com
website 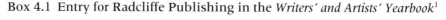www.radcliffe-oxford.com

Directors Andrew Bax (managing), Gill Nineham (editorial), Margaret McKeown (financial), Gregory Moxon (marketing)

Primary care, child health, palliative care, nursing, pharmacy, dentistry, healthcare organisation and management. Founded 1987.

Your book proposal needs to be convincing in the following ways.

- You and the other authors or editor are the right people to be writing or editing it – perhaps well known for your specialisms, providing the right perspectives, with experience of writing.
- The fields that you will be covering are pertinent to the potential readership and within the scope of the authors' or editor's expertise.
- Increased sales will result from the book being relevant to as many potential readership groups as possible. This could be as a textbook for undergraduate or postgraduate courses, an integral part of continuing professional development for health and social care staff groups, an updating of the application of new legal requirements or policy for managers and employers, or of special interest to health and social care staff developing new knowledge and skills for particular roles, etc.
- There is room for a new book in the specified area. The book proposal describes the competition and justifies why the proposed book is superior to, different from or complements those already available.
- Give the book as wide an appeal as possible for a varied potential readership without losing its specific appeal for the needs of particular readers.
- Focus on niche areas or write on popular topics to boost potential sales. When

you describe whether similar books already exist, explain how yours is better, different or complementary.

Look at publishers' websites for their guidance on whether book proposals are welcome, and if so how they should be constructed. Some examples are given in Box 4.2.

Before opting for a particular publisher, check out what other books they publish in your area of interest, so that you can be sure they are an appropriate choice and do not list a book just like your proposed one. You can always phone up the contact person at a particular publishing house as stated in the *Writers' and Artists' Yearbook.*[1] You could talk though the possibility of submitting a book proposal, the scope of the book and your intended readership, to establish how interested the publisher might be and what detail they want you to submit.

Box 4.2 Examples of guidance for various publishers of books for health and social care professions

1 Elsevier Science

The Health Sciences Division publishes in the broad areas of:

- nursing, midwifery and health visiting
- dentistry
- pharmacy
- other allied health fields
- complementary therapies
- textbooks for medical students or junior trainees
- professional and reference books for specialist doctors.

The information about preparing a publication proposal relating to nursing, midwifery and health visiting advises you to prepare your own submission or download a standard proposal form. The name and contact details of the publishing director are given so that you can discuss your ideas with them before preparing a detailed book proposal, and ensure that a similar book is not already in the pipeline.

The outline of the book proposal should include:

- a working title – as explicit as possible
- aims and scope – why it is being written, why it is needed, what it will cover, what is special about the approach, what is special about the style, what is special about the authors and/or editors
- target market (the group for whom it is intended) and secondary markets (others who may be interested)
- contents – about 30–100 words per chapter as a synopsis of what will be included with the main subheadings, and the chapters listed in sequence
- approximate number of words
- illustrations and tables – their content and purpose
- competing and complementary books – noting how your proposed book differs from them
- author(s) or editor(s) – a brief CV for each, and a provisional list of contributors (but there is no need to have approached them at this stage)

- sample chapter of around 3000–4000 words to show the level, approach and style of the book.

http://intl.elsevierhealth.com/author/quest2a_frames.cfm

2 Oxford University Press

New book suggestions and proposals are welcomed. You are invited to approach the appropriate editor by email or telephone to discuss whether your proposal is likely to fit with their publishing programme.

Similar information about structuring the book proposal is given to that for Elsevier above.

www.oup.co.uk/academic/medicine/editorial/

3 Routledge

Routledge are keen to consider proposals for new books. They suggest that a proposal should be 3–4 pages in length, accompanied by sample chapters or a draft manuscript, and authors'/editors' CVs. They require a similar content to the book proposal as Elsevier do (*see* above and their website). The guidance about word length states that most of their books are 80,000–100,000 words. State when you will deliver your typescript.

www.routledge.com/proposal.asp

Look at the publisher's peer-reviewer form to do a final check that your draft book proposal has addressed all of the publisher's issues. A publisher will usually check the viability of a book proposal with two or three independent referees who know the field. They know what new books might be required and may have heard of other similar books already in the publication process. Look at the website of the publisher you are targeting to see if a book-proposal review form can be downloaded, or maybe ring one of the editorial contacts listed and ask for one. Then make sure that your draft book proposal covers all of the areas of enquiry on the peer-review form satisfactorily.

Prepare several drafts of your book proposal before submitting it. Novice writers tend to be satisfied with early versions of their work, whether that is the book proposal or the actual chapters. More experienced authors are often more exacting and expect to redraft versions of their work as many as ten times until they are satisfied with the final product.

Before you submit the book proposal to your selected publisher, look at it with critical eyes. Are some proposed chapters weaker than others and could they be strengthened? Is there a good balance between theory and application? Could you widen the book's appeal to an international readership by maybe expanding the case studies while retaining its relevance to your immediate target groups?

As you redraft your book proposal, integrate ideas and suggestions from any co-authors or your mentor, or others in the field. If a publisher turns down your proposal, try to find out why and consider whether their comments are relevant to your concept of the book, and again redraft accordingly to improve the proposal. Think about the planned book when you are driving in the car, on country walks, in bed or in the bath. Capture those creative ideas by jotting down your thoughts, and revise the proposal.

The example of a book proposal in Box 4.3 is the original proposal for this book. Bear in mind as you scrutinise it that the two main authors, Ruth and Gill, were already well-established writers and well known to the publishing house, Radcliffe Publishing Ltd. The other two co-authors, who have little published work to their credit, were part of the writing team because of their key expertise in relation to the process of publishing. Michele was recruited as a chapter contributor to write about the role of literary agents because none of the four co-authors had personal experience of agents. The publishing house had already expressed an interest in commissioning such a book at a preliminary brainstorming meeting with some of their established writers. The example of the contents of the proposal given here in Box 4.3 represents the minimum that would be included.

If you are not an established writer and any of your co-authors are also unknown, you will need to demonstrate that you can write well and in the style that the publisher usually adopts. Some publishers expect at least one chapter to be submitted with the book proposal, and this sample chapter might be about 10% of the word count of the finished book manuscript (*see* Box 4.2). If this is the first chapter, that has the additional advantage of setting the scene for the book and providing more information for the potential publisher and their peer reviewers about whether your book proposal is well justified. If you are intending the book to be really creative or different from other competitive or complementary ones, supply a typical chapter to show why your format is exciting.

Finalising practical details within your book proposal

As well as agreeing the structure of the book proposal to convince your chosen publishing house to commission you, there are practical details that you and your co-authors or co-editors will need to agree with you, unless you're going solo. One essential agreement concerns the format, language and style that you will use in the book – and this will be reflected in the content of the book proposal. For instance, it includes the extent to which you use jargon, abbreviations, 'you' or 'we' or 'I' or the third person, the inclusion of case studies and their nature, the balance between theory and practical material, the extent of similarity in the structure of each chapter, etc.

Discuss and agree a realistic timescale for submitting the final manuscript. Allow for the publisher organising the peer review of your book proposal. Consider what else is going on in your life – with your family or at work – and your career pathway that might prevent you from writing to an ideal timescale. Try to match your manuscript submission to the timings of any regulations or legislation for which the book is important. There is no point in rushing the writing before new policy changes so that the book is already noticeably out of date on the day it is published. On the other hand, you should avoid delaying writing and submitting the manuscript when profound changes take place. If your book is not available, potential readers cannot buy it and must struggle to understand or apply things themselves. Discuss important timings with the publisher so that they can determine whether it is worth fast-tracking your manuscript, or possible to do so, when they are deciding whether to commission the book.

You may have a guide from the publisher concerning the word count of their usual published books and whether that includes indexing, contents, preface, etc. Bear this word count in mind when you agree the approximate word count of each chapter with whoever is the lead writer for that chapter. This will help you to achieve a balance between chapters from the beginning. One of you will be writing the typical draft chapter to append to the book proposal, too – in the format and style you have all agreed (*see* Chapter 8).

Another practical detail to fix between co-authors and co-editors is how they will share the royalties from writing the book – or the fee if the publisher pays a fee up front or on publication. The book proposal in Box 4.3 shows that the share of royalties reflected the proportion of time and effort that each writer was likely to spend on writing their part of the book manuscript, and the lead role that Ruth would take as editor of the whole typescript – putting the proposal together, proof checking and book promotion, collating the co-authors' mini-CVs, etc.

Box 4.3 Example of a book proposal

How to Succeed series: Publishing a book

Ruth Chambers, contact details: address/email/telephone
Gill Wakley, contact details: address/email/telephone
Gill Nineham, contact details: address/email/telephone
Gregory Moxon, contact details: address/email/telephone
Michele Topham, contact details: address/email/telephone
Royalties 10% for first 1000 books sold, 12.5% thereafter
Ruth C 50%, Gill W 30%, Gill N 10%, Gregory M 10% [Gregory M/Gill N royalties to be diverted to a charitable fund]
Chapter contributors £100 cheque or £150 book tokens
Submission date 31-1-06

1 The outline

1.1 Title: Publishing a book

1.2 Target market

Anyone writing for health and social care personnel, including doctors and other health and social care professionals, and managers/support staff and academics. The text will be generalisable to sectors other than health and social care.

1.3 Aims and scope

Why is the book being written?

To help those who are contemplating writing a book, or whose first attempts have not been successful.

Why is it needed?

Many people waste a great deal of time thinking about writing a book and not proceeding, or are put off by not knowing how to go about it. If readers develop more knowledge and skills in writing a book proposal and then a book, they should be able to target their efforts at writing more exactly and

---

will be more likely to succeed in producing a book that addresses the potential readership's needs and sells well.

What will it cover?

Please see chapter contents.

How much depth?

As detailed as necessary to enable the reader to understand the context, how to do it and lots of tips for more effective writing.

1.4 What is special about the style?

All writing will be in a clear and practical style. The reader will feel that this has been written by people who are experienced in writing and are familiar with the reality of struggling to plan, prepare and then undertake the writing of a book – in competitive fields.

1.5 What is special about the approach?

a) The practical style with tips and advice that can be integrated into the reader's own field or circumstances.

b) The book will encourage the reader to think more widely about writing – and to gauge the chances of achieving their vision for a best-selling book more realistically.

c) The positive and logical approach to writing books – showing how to do it.

d) The book will help the reader to learn from their writing experience, and to consider the future whether or not their first book proposal is successful – for example, how else the effort and investment spent on preparation can be utilised, or how else they can develop a different book proposal if the first book proposal submission is unsuccessful.

1.6 Content

Chapter 1. Why write a book?

- You know a lot/want to share it.
- The challenge – you always wanted to write.
- You write articles and want to progress to a book.
- A 'legacy.'
- It's expected in your role.
- Academic profile – PhD, etc. (but books rank lower in the RAE than peer-reviewed journal papers).
- You love your own thinking, so everyone else will, too.
- To influence national debate – no one else interrupts as they can when you're talking.
- You're not good at talking, so write instead.
- Someone pays you to do it.
- Asked by a publisher.

3500 words
Ruth C

Chapter 2. When and what to write

- Depends on your reason.
- Any time in your career – or middle/end – but don't procrastinate.

- A series, ongoing.
- After a project ceases – disseminate findings of the project.
- While you're setting up a project, and enthusiastic.
- When trying to pass on information and evidence.

2500 words
Ruth C/Gill W

Chapter 3. In what capacity will you be writing?

- Pros and cons of being an author, a co-author or an editor.
- If an author, finding co-author(s). What will it take for you to be able to work together? How can you assess whether you can work together as co-authors? Writing with someone you don't know well.
- If an editor, what editing power will you have?
- If an editor, will you contribute chapters, too?
- Write with others to 'mentor you.'
- Write a chapter or two in someone else's book.
- If you're the lead, how do you decide which contributors to invite to do what?
- Why not write articles instead of a book (easier and more lucrative)?
- Original material versus adapting others' ideas.
- Expert or commentator?

3500 words
Ruth C

Chapter 4. How to write a convincing book proposal

- Do market research – get justification for book, help shape book.
- Ask friends/colleagues how they did it.
- Prepare a book proposal using a template from colleague/publisher.
- Find publisher. Then submit proposal to publisher, send example chapters or published articles – demonstrate ability, match to likely readership, write proposal as a group of writers so that there are fewer blind spots.
- Make several drafts of book proposal – write down ideas to integrate into it (in bed/in the bath).
- Suggest realistic deadline for submission – match to timings of any regulations/legislation for which book is important.
- Word count.
- Royalties – suggest percentage.
- Literary agent – necessary? How to find one. Fees.

Getting your proposal accepted

- Justify market need – demonstrate likely sales to which readership groups (academic courses, general public, professions).
- Make appeal as wide as possible without losing specific appeal to main readership groups.
- Focus on niches or write on popular topics – describe whether similar books are already on market, and if so why yours is better/different.

4500 words
Ruth C

Chapter 5. Choosing a publisher

- Match to readership.
- Why it matters: publishers specialising in different areas, targeting their marketing/promotion, fit with profile, some only publish academic books, etc.
- Difference between professional and trade publishing.
- Marketing that publisher does – unsolicited mailings, bulk sales.
- Reliability.
- Timescale for publishing process.
- Guaranteed publication?
- Vanity publishing.

3000 words
Gill W

Chapter 6. Having a literary agent

- What do literary agents do?
- When is it worth getting a literary agent?
- How can you find a literary agent?
- How do you know the literary agent is the right one for you?

2500 words
Michele T

Chapter 7. Writing the book

- Making time – meeting deadlines.
- Making time for writing: early in morning/late at night.
- Clear timetable.
- Go away for a few days?
- Write on the train.
- Gather material for months beforehand.
- Carry a notebook with you and make jottings.
- Deadlines – know and keep to them (submission, copy-editor deadlines, etc.).
- Be available to copy editor and publisher to answer queries promptly so as not to hold up the process.
- Self-discipline; ways of getting down to work; rewards.
- What to do when you're stuck.
- Find a coach or buddy to keep you at it, take an interest and encourage you.
- Peer – point out gaps.
- Arranging a foreword – famous person, use as quotes in advertising literature.
- Someone to proofread.

5000 words
Gill W

Chapter 8. Style

- Decide on the format.
- Use case studies/boxes to break up the text.
- Anecdotes: pros and cons.

- Match any publisher requirements (e.g. humour, style).
- Select jokes, cartoons/illustrations to enhance text/reflect style.
- Avoid jargon.
- Describe new concepts, abbreviations, etc. in full the first time alluded to.
- Keep to your style – harmonise styles if different writers write various chapters – have seamless editing throughout.
- Agree on use of 'you', 'we', 'one' or 'I' throughout.
- References; sources of evidence for statements.
- Personal view or evidence for text?

3000 words
Gill W

Chapter 9. The publisher's side: editorial and production

- Do algorithm of pathway from submission of book proposal to publication.
- What the publisher looks for in book proposal.
- Peer review of book proposal.
- How book proposal fits with other published books or books in press – own company and other publishers.
- Deadlines – importance of meeting them.
- Sticking to the remit of the book proposal – word length, style, content, authorship.
- Copy-editing process.
- Paper versus electronic publication.
- Translation into foreign languages.
- Book fairs.
- The contract.
- What the authors get – free books, discount on books, profile.
- Revisions to proof of manuscript (keep them minor, check websites, etc.).

3500 words
Gill N

Chapter 10. The publisher's side: finance, marketing and promotion

- Finance – behind-the-scenes costings.
- The marketing meeting – the title, the likely market.
- Royalties – how much, proportion of management costs, from overseas rights.
- Profit – how much is a minimum.
- Promotion – who does what, what authors can do to help.
- What publisher wants in book-promotion questionnaire.
- Publish extracts of book and advertise it.
- Offer prize of free books to promote it in national press.
- Get authors interested in using book on courses or in their work.
- Sales – minimum to expect in order to be viable, pushing up sales.

2500 words
Gregory M

Chapter 11. Improving your writing technique
- Read reviews of book – reflect and consider where reviewers' opinions differ.
- Join writers' association – critique each others' work.
- Do reviews of others' books for national press.
- Go on a writing course (academic, creative).
- Experiment with other types of writing (articles, etc.).
- Experiment with different styles (simple, academic).

2500 words
Ruth C

Sources of help Information about publishers; websites

1.7 Approximate words
About 40,000 words.

1.8 Illustrations and tables
Five illustrations drawn by John Barker.

2 Competing or complementary books

Cormack DFS. *Writing for Health Care Professions.* Oxford: Blackwell Scientific Publications; 1994.
Spicer R. *How to Publish a Book.* 2nd ed. Plymouth: How To Books; 1995.
Fraser J. *How to Publish in Biomedicine.* Oxford: Radcliffe Medical Press; 1997.
Cook R. *The Writer's Manual.* Oxford: Radcliffe Medical Press; 1999.
Albert T. *Winning the Publications Game.* 2nd ed. Oxford: Radcliffe Medical Press; 2000.

3 About the authors

Brief biographies of each author and chapter contributor.

If you look closely you will see that the final book content does differ from that indicated by our book proposal in Box 4.3. Some publishers are more flexible than others in the extent to which they allow authors to divert from the agreed book proposal.

Reference

1 Pratchett T. *Writers' and Artists' Yearbook 2006.* London: A & C Black; 2005.

Chapter 5

Choosing a publisher

Gill Wakley

Just as you do not wander through life hoping that you will win the jackpot on the lottery to solve your financial problems, do not wait for a publisher to approach you if you want to write a book. Get out there and look for one. Do not write the book and send it to a publisher you have picked out with a pin. Do your research, and then prepare a book proposal (*see* Chapter 4) and sample chapters to send to your carefully selected choice of publisher. Occasionally, a publisher will approach you. An editor or director has become aware of your writing in journals on a subject and the publishing house has a gap that they would like filled. Rejoice, and then prepare your book proposal.

Advice from established authors

If you know people who have had books published, ask for their advice. Unless they are in direct competition with you with a similar book, they will generally be happy to give their advice and opinions. They may be able to tell you about books in the pipeline that might be competing against your intended one as well.

Keep in mind the characteristics of the person you are asking. If he or she is known to be a rigid thinker, not a team player, with egocentric or eccentric ideas, the advice may not be applicable to you. People like that often think that they can write excellent books, but fail to have the audience or the publisher's editor in mind as they write. Others get on well with all the publishers they use – they are the authors who address the publishers' requirements, remembering to check that they have sent everything needed, getting their copy of the manuscript in on time and turning the queries and proofs around quickly. If one of these paragons has had difficulties with a specific publisher, listen carefully. Bear in mind that it may just have been a clash of personalities with a specific editor – but might you get that one, too?

Even if you receive a specific recommendation, it is wise to do your own research on that publisher's catalogue and requirements.

Publishing with the publishing arm of an organisation

You are likely to belong to an organisation such as a Royal College, Institute or Society that represents your specialty. Most of the larger ones publish books, but may contract out the work to a publishing house. Look at their output. Much of it will consist of reports of symposia, or commissioned work for members or collected articles from the journal(s) that they publish. If you are involved in committee or development work for your College or Society, you may be involved in the preparation of reports and have cut your teeth on how the process functions in a low-risk situation.

You do not need to belong to an organisation to use their publishing arm (*see* Box 5.1).

Box 5.1 Examples of the publishing arm of organisations

1 RSM Press is the publishing arm of the Royal Society of Medicine, a postgraduate medical society with a multidisciplinary and multiprofessional membership. It publishes books and journals for the medical profession and professionals working in related fields. Authors need to approach the managing director with any book proposal.
2 The Pharmaceutical Press is the publications division of the Royal Pharmaceutical Society of Great Britain. It produces books, journals and related digital products on pharmacy, pharmaceutical sciences and other related disciplines. The website has easy-to-find resources for authors, and can be found at www.pharmpress.com
3 BMJ Books are now part of Blackwells Publishers. Blackwells have a medical list for medical students, hospital medicine and some specialised areas such as sports medicine, but currently have no family practice list. They have a separate list for professions allied to medicine (e.g. nursing, health and social care, dietetics, pharmacy and dentistry).
4 The Royal College of General Practitioners publishes much of its own output of advice, symposium reports, guidance papers, etc. It will accept manuscript proposals relevant to primary care. The Editor of College Publications and other professionals (usually two) with special interests assess Occasional Papers. Other books may be submitted as proposals with a sample chapter, but preferably as a full-length text. They are also subject to assessment by expert referees. Further details can be found at www.rcgp.org.uk/default.aspx?page=618

Charitable organisation publishing

Many charities publish leaflets and information for their users. Some of them also publish books and may be interested in one on a subject relevant to their membership. For example, a book on handling and moving people with back pain and disabilities might appeal to several charities involved with caring for people with these problems. Usually they will only be interested in books for the public, but some, like the Family Planning Association, also publish books of interest to professionals. Your target readership must be specific to the interests of the charity. They may have precise requirements for layout and format, so you need to be flexible in the way you write to match their target audience. Do your own research about their requirements before writing your book proposal.

Finding a publisher from scratch

You could use a reference source either in a library or on the Internet to look for information about all the publishers. So many publishers, so little time! Instead, look at the non-fiction books on your bookshelves, particularly those that you have bought yourself and have read and used. These are likely to be on your subject of interest and indicate the publishers in your field. Make a list of the publishers that seem like possibilities.

Then look at the type of book that those publishers produce. Is it an atlas with pictures, a revision aid, or an exploration of the impact of legislation change? Mark on your list which publishers match the type of book that you have in mind. If you have been favourably impressed by the layout and organisation of a book, give them a star.

Now you have a shortlist to research. Look first at their addresses. The bigger publishers will have several offices in different countries, usually because they have taken over other publishing houses (*see* the example in Box 5.2).

Box 5.2 Example of confusion and multiplicity

Elsevier (itself part of the Reed Business Group) has offices in Amsterdam (its head office), London, Oxford, Shannon, Paris, Munich, New York, Chicago, Boston, Philadelphia, San Diego, St Louis, Toronto, Rio de Janeiro, Singapore, Sydney, Tokyo and Beijing.

Elsevier's medical imprints include:

- Academic Press
- Baillière Tindall
- BC Decker
- Butterworth-Heinemann
- Churchill Livingston
- GW Medical Publishing
- Hanley & Belfus
- Mosby
- Saunders and Wolfe.

Look to see which subsidiary has an office in which country. If the publishing house has no editorial base in your country, think again. Although much of your communication can be by email, do you really want to have to send your completed manuscript to Melbourne or Chicago? You may have to send it by overseas post if you live in the British Virgin Isles, but most of us are luckier and have more local publishing offices. Next, look up the publisher's website and inspect their catalogue or list. If you cannot find one, they may have gone out of business, or been taken over by another publishing house (a frequent occurrence).

The publisher's list

Look first at the number and range of books in their catalogue. It will vary enormously between publishers, from a small list of 20–30 books to thousands. Similarly, the range of the list will vary from a few subjects to many hundred. It is difficult to know whether to opt for a large or small publisher. Some of the large publishers will have several different imprints (examples are shown in Box 5.3), and you could spend hours trying to choose between them.

Box 5.3 Publishers with different imprints

A publisher well known for medical books is Lippincott Williams & Wilkins. They are part of Wolters Kluer Publishing, with other publishers specialising in different subjects.

Taylor & Francis Books has a catalogue of medical, biomedical and pharmaceutical science books, published by the following individual publishers:

- Taylor & Francis
- Marcel Dekker
- Routledge
- Martin Dunitz
- Parthenon Publishing
- CRC Press publications.

The main website (www.ebookstore.tandf.co.uk/html/index.asp) has useful information for potential authors and a very wide-ranging list of titles.

At least the choice is easier with a smaller to medium-sized publisher whose list you know includes the kind of books you like and could emulate – or revolutionise! The Radcliffe Publishing website (www.radcliffe-oxford.com/aboutrmp.htm) gives information about their business and a list of their fields of interest, as well as a downloadable catalogue. Their e-bulletin tells you who to contact to discuss writing a book for their list (tip: it is Gill Nineham).

Some smaller publishers may have restricted interests. For example, despite its grand-sounding name, Advanced Medical Publishing only covers radiation oncology and diagnostic radiology. Beaconsfield Publishers produce only two or three books a year and of their list of 39 books, 21 are on homeopathy. CAB International has a list on public health and communicable diseases, human nutrition and food science. Fine if that is your field.

Too small a publisher and it may not have the facilities you need. Too big and it may be too impersonal (*see* Box 5.4).

Box 5.4 Advantages and disadvantages of small and large publishing houses

For	*Against*
The small business	
A more personal touch from the editor	The editor may be autocratic and overbearing. If you do not get on, there is no one else who could take over as editor. The small business may be taken over by a larger one
Helps me more	Unless there are house guidelines, you are dependent on the editor's inclination and interest
May be quicker	Depending on how many other books the editor is handling. Peaks and troughs are less easy to manage with fewer staff
More at stake in making sure that my book is successful	They may have fewer contacts and contracts with booksellers. Fewer staff might mean that there is no one available to push your book
More likely to accept innovative ideas	Finance is more at risk, so you may be less likely to get your book proposal accepted unless you convince them that it is a winner
Easy to identify what will interest them	Do not confuse a legitimate small publisher with a vanity press. If they ask you to pay a fee or list people who will buy your book, back off
Large publishing house	
Identifiable editor dealing with only a few authors	The editor may change, possibly several times, during the preparation of your book
Will have the experience to help me more	The editor may be as new as you
Will be quicker	Your editor may have to fight with others to get a place on the printing schedule
Will have many contacts with organisations, bookshops, etc. for good sales	Unless your editor is convincing, the salesperson may have less interest in pushing your book compared with others on the list
Has the finance to take a risk with an innovative format	Depends on the policy of the business
Wide list, so likely to take my book	May already have sufficient books on that subject and be unwilling to add to them

Requirements for authors

If the website contains the type of book that you want to write, or have started writing, look at their requirements for authors. Some have printed forms that you need to complete. Others just ask you to contact the editor or managing director for a chat. The ease with which you can obtain information about submitting a book varies, too.

You may have narrowed it down on your previous searches and found that Manson Publishing, for instance, issues books for professionals and students in medicine, veterinary medicine and the sciences. They say that they specialise in highly illustrated books for study and reference, produced in full colour. They have an office in London. You decide that this publisher is just what you want for your book, which includes lots of colour photographs, and you discover a quick and clear website with instructions for potential authors at www.manson-publishing.co.uk.

Alternatively, you want to go for one of the prestigious or well-established imprints on the recommendation of a friend. Oxford University Press has a large list on varied subjects and has offices in both the UK and the USA. General advice on submissions is available at www.oup.co.uk/academic/medicine/editorial/, but the Acrobat files on support and guidelines for authors are less easy to find. Another author recommends McGraw Hill (www.mcgraw-hill.com), based in New York. Their list also contains many classic textbooks. The instructions to authors sound long-winded and discursive. Perhaps the slightly old-fashioned approach might suit your serious textbook better.

Alternatively, you may be looking for a new and keen publisher and have identified TFM (www.tfmpublishing.co.uk), who say that their company is eager to build its book list and can offer all the support and guidance that an author will need to take an idea or manuscript through to a finished book. You look at their very small list of 27 books and think that it appears very eclectic and they must be dying to have your book. You note that they ask for a CV of the author along with an outline of the book, a couple of sample chapters if these are ready, the book's unique selling points and its likely market by email. You hardly notice their caveat that there are many hopeful authors seeking a publisher to take on their project, and not all approaches can be taken on.

Being rejected

When the publisher writes back to say that your proposed book is not suitable, you feel devastated. However, do not take it personally. It may be that you chose the wrong publisher, or the wrong time. Some publishers will helpfully tell you why they and their independent peer reviewers rejected it. If it does not match their list, this may tell you that your research was not thorough enough and the target was incorrect. You may not have identified competing books, or made yours different enough. Do your research again and try again.

Self-publishing

Cutting out the middleman and doing it yourself sounds a good idea until you think about all that is involved. You may have written your thesis to the specifications of your university and had five copies bound, but that is a far cry from planning, writing, formatting, printing and binding large numbers of books. Then you have to market them without the contacts that publishers build up.

If you wrote a handbook to go with a course, you may have printed and ring-bound perhaps 20 to 200 copies. These you have given away, or rather you have built the cost into the price of the course. Printing for profit and persuading people to buy 200 copies is more complicated.

Reasons for considering self-publishing

Your book may be on a little known subject or one of limited interest – perhaps a history of a local hospital that is now closed – and you are certain that the number of copies sold will be small. You are unlikely to find a publisher under these circumstances, and self-publishing may appeal to you. Look at the alternatives to doing it all yourself. A university or local society may be willing to help with publication (at a cost!).

You may be absolutely convinced that there will be a market for your book, even if the publishers you have approached have declined to accept it, saying that the market for it is limited or that there are too many similar books available already. Susan went ahead in this way, as described in Box 5.5, with a successful outcome, although such happy endings rarely occur.

Box 5.5 Going it alone with self-publishing

Susan approached Radcliffe Publishing with a book proposal that she felt could not fail to be a big seller. Unfortunately for Susan, the publisher had already commissioned a book with a similar content, and although they liked the book suggestion they did not accept the proposal. Susan went ahead with self-publishing, and at the same time wrote several articles targeted at her potential readership in a medical careers supplement. A year or two later, she had sold more than 750 copies herself and Radcliffe accepted her revised book proposal the second time round, when there was no competitive book in the offing.[1]

If you want to write a book or a resource that will need very frequent updating, think about using a website rather than a book, or putting an e-book on a website. Unless you charge people per view, it will not make any money, but it is easy to update provided that you spend the time on it (and you would have to anyway).

Necessities

The most important commodities are plenty of time and some willing helpers. Experience with printing many copies of a handbook, course notes or similar publications helps. Look at books to see the layout (*see also* Chapter 7) and learn about how and what to put on alternate pages. You need an ISBN[2] – an International Standard Book Number. Without an ISBN, your book will not be included in bibliographies or book lists.

If you are doing the printing yourself, a heavy-duty laser printer is essential. It has to cope with the quality of the print and collating the pages, so that it can print a book at a time. You can learn bookbinding, or go to a commercial source (obviously more expensive). You could use spiral binding, but this only looks suitable on a workbook or something that is not intended to last for long. Also, the title on spiral bound books is difficult to read when placed on shelves in libraries or bookshops, and may therefore decrease potential sales and readers. Then you need to market it.

Paying to be published

So-called 'vanity publishing' is a great money-spinner for the companies doing it. Many websites offer help with 'self-publishing', and some small publishers are making money at your expense. If the ISBN belongs to the company, this is not 'self-publishing.' Some businesses will publish the book at no cost to yourself with the proviso that they produce large numbers of books that they sell to all your relatives and friends (you will need lots of these). Others actually charge you to publish the book.

If you think your book is worth publishing, spend the time looking for a proper publisher who will pay you royalties and market your book skilfully. There is little money to be made in non-fiction writing, but you should not have to pay for it yourself if your writing is worth publishing.

References

1 Kersley S. *Prescription for Change*. Oxford: Radcliffe Publishing; 2006.
2 www.isbn-international.org/en/howtoget.html

Chapter 6

Having a literary agent

Michele Topham

What do literary agents do?

The word *agent* can still conjure up the image of a man with an astrakhan coat and a fat cigar, pushing up fees to cover his 10%. However, the right literary agent can make both the author's and the publisher's lives easier. A literary agent is a link between author and publisher – a negotiator, a facilitator, and occasionally a buffer.

Publishing is a sociable industry. Publishers and literary agents are communicators and networkers. An agent will build a network of publishing contacts which an author, who is busy maintaining his or her own career, cannot realistically hope to do. They also have pulling power – an agent with a client list of authors is more powerful than one author on his or her own, however valuable. A publisher is less likely to jeopardise their relationship with an agent who looks after a number of authors than with one individual author.

An agent will have accumulated experience of publishing terms, industry conditions and problem solving. A new author with an agent has access to knowledge which they would not otherwise have.

The literary agent's job may begin with advising you on the shape of your book proposal. You may have a good knowledge of your subject, but not have developed the skills required to summarise your theories and shape them into an accessible presentation for publishers. Publishers have limited time in which to read through submitted proposals from new authors, and may dismiss a proposal that might, if shaped by an experienced hand, be more instantly appealing. There is no cut-out-and-keep formula for writing a book proposal, but a literary agent has experience of what publishers need to see and can cast a fresh and objective eye over what you have written.

When it comes to finding a publisher for your proposed book, an agent will know, from their accumulated experience and access to the publishing network, which are the best and most likely publishers and editors for that book. You may know of one or two publishers of books in your field, but an agent will know of more. Having a greater number of potential publishers increases the possibility of your book being published, and of it being published by the best publisher for you on the best possible financial terms.

There is a two-way street between publishers and agents. You may propose a book and your agent will take it to a publisher. Alternatively, a publisher may have a particular book in mind which they would like to publish, and they will know which literary agents to approach in order to interest likely authors. If you are on an agent's client list, some of the future books that you write will not necessarily be ones you had thought of yourself initially.

Your agent may also suggest likely projects and will advise you on what books may work best for you and when. If you are hoping to write a number of books, it is useful to have a 'career adviser' to help you plan. This is a function that your friendly and supportive agent can fulfil.

With fiction, the creative process is different. Only you can tell your story, and an agent or editor cannot suggest what you should write. However, an agent who shares your love of a particular kind of fiction can offer impartial advice when you are stuck on a plot or stylistic matter – objective scrutiny can draw you away from all kinds of writer's block. Whatever kind of fiction you write, your agent will know what fiction editors are looking for and what is selling in bookshops. If your novel is not finding its mark, they will know when it is time to put it back in your bottom drawer and move on to the next book.

Once your agent has happily found a publisher for your book, they will negotiate your contract, and this is where you benefit from their being able to exercise their strength to the power of many authors, rather than your strength to the power of one. The agency will have agreed 'boilerplate' terms – a set of basic contract terms which publishers agree to use for that agency's authors, which will be based on the agency's knowledge of the fairest available terms and conditions of a book contract. Just as the agent has knowledge of a broad number and range of publishers, so they will have knowledge and experience of the best terms, from the size of the advance, the range of royalties and the number of rights (for instance, for different formats and territories) to the finer details of late-delivery penalty clauses, and the get-out clause which comes into play when your book is no longer selling. If you do not have experience of book contracts, a publisher is not likely to give anything away, but they will appreciate that the agent knows the full value of your book.

A standard contract between a publisher and an author is likely to include all possible rights. However, an agent may feel that the original publisher is not best placed to produce the book in all those formats and territories, and will argue that they should retain them on your behalf. The agent will either have colleagues who will sell those rights to the best secondary publishers (for paperback editions, translation, etc.) and producers (for film, television and radio), or will have an established relationship with other agents or agencies who will work on a commission split to sell your book further afield. Commission on those sales is always, of necessity, more than commission for local sales.

Once contracts have been signed, you will be feeling that this is your bit, and that you can settle down and write the planned book and look forward to publication day. However, there are potential problems in the publishing process. Slow authors, slow publishers, a change of editor, lack of communication at key moments and fear of looming deadlines are all frequent occurrences. Publishers are busy and multitask, whereas authors are out there on their own, without colleagues to consult. Your agent will have a relationship both with you and with your publisher, and will have past experience of the pitfalls of the publishing process and what it takes to bridge them. They will be your adviser and champion and even, on a lonely day at your desk, someone at the other end of the phone to cheer you up when you are stuck.

There are many things to keep an eye on once the book has been published. You may wonder why your book has not hit the best-seller list, nor been feted in the *Sunday Times*. Your agent will look at what might be the reasons. They can, if appropriate, chase your publisher and ask them to increase publicity, or to increase their print run or rally their sales force. Or they can gently explain to you that your market is just not the one which attracts the *Sunday Times* readership or the big-spending public.

Sales figures may be one of the mysteries of your annual or bi-annual royalty statement. Your agent will check statements and keep a record of the book's sales history. They will pursue anomalies (possible erroneous accounting, royalty rates, unexpectedly large sales to discount sources) and bring their power to bear on the publishers in any dispute.

They will also monitor any decline in book sales. When sales have fallen, it may be that your book has reached the end of its useful time with your publisher. Your agent will request a reversion of the publisher's rights to you, having at contract stage negotiated a clause which prevents the publisher from sitting on rights if the book is not selling. A good agent will not let an out-of-print book go out of sight, and will pursue any potential for reprints and revised editions.

However, your agent does not focus on just one book but on the whole of your writing career, and will always look for suitable new projects and be realistic about your suggestions and plans. Many agents will arrange opportunities in complementary media, such as radio, television and journalism. Their network will extend beyond book publishing, and could provide you with interesting and valuable additions to your writing output.

Is it worth having an agent?

Consider what a literary agent does, and then consider whether you need any or all of those services. Agents take commission on all authors' earnings which have been negotiated by them, so you must remember that you will be paying for their services and balance that payment against what you may gain.

There are a number of good reasons why it might not be useful or appropriate to involve a literary agent.

- There may be a limited number of publishers specialising in your kind of book.
- You may have been approached to write your book by a publisher who has already developed the proposal to an advanced stage. It is unlikely that they will agree to higher terms for a project they have developed themselves.
- Some specialist publishers have fixed terms and are unable (or unwilling) to change, so contracts are not negotiable.
- Your book may be part of a series and, for practical reasons, all texts have to conform to a particular format and all authors will receive the same terms.
- You may only plan to write one book in your career, which you feel you have the capacity to sell effectively yourself.
- You may feel that you have the time and energy to act as your own agent, enjoying the challenge and saving yourself the commission.

In all these instances, it may be difficult for a literary agent to bring anything extra to the relationship between you and your publisher.

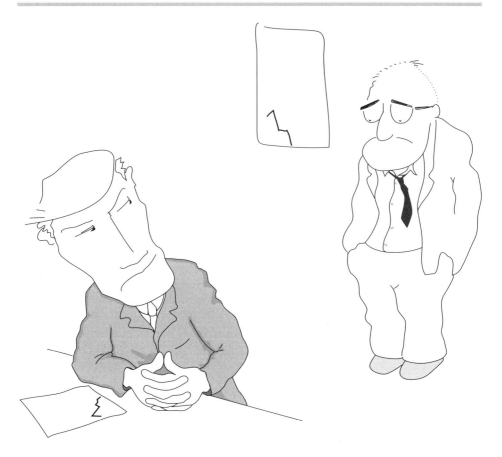

When I said your books were selling like hot cakes, what I meant was that no-one will buy any quantities for fear of getting their fingers burnt.

How do you find a literary agent?

Guidebook research and word of mouth are the most productive ways of finding an agent. The two most widely read guidebooks are *The Writer's Handbook*[1] and the *Writers' and Artists' Yearbook*.[2] They are updated annually and contain the names and addresses of agents (as well as publishers and other related bodies) and a small amount of detail about the agencies' specialist subjects and some of the authors they represent. *The Writer's Handbook* has a useful subject index at the back, which is worth reading through to find out who is listed under your particular subject or subjects. The *Writers' and Artists' Yearbook* contains essays on matters of interest to writers.

There is also an increasing number of Internet sites that list literary agents, some of which also give details of their specialist subjects. Many literary agents have websites which give details about themselves and their clients. The website will give you an idea of whether they are the kind of agency that might suit you.

If you are not shy about telling people that you are writing a book, ask likely friends and colleagues if they know of any literary agents. If you are a member of an academic organisation and your book relates to your academic work, ask colleagues in the common room. Just as you may meet your partner through friends or colleagues who know you and your habits, so you may meet your agent through friends and colleagues who share your interests and work experience.

The right literary agent for you

If someone has recommended an agent, you will have a certain amount of confidence in them. You will be fairly sure that their practices are good and that they are respected by publishers and writers alike. If they are already representing one of your colleagues, you will know that they have experience in your field.

If instead you are cold-calling agents, you should check their credentials. Check the guidebooks and check the authors they already represent. The agent needs to be familiar with your kind of book in order to appreciate its possibilities and approach the right publishers. Check the agency terms before you approach them. Most agents have uniform terms, but some will have different ways of operating.

Once you have selected an agent or agents you think may be suitable, write to them, sending your CV, the synopsis of your book and some sample chapters. You may be an excellent writer but, just as there may be certain writers whose books you buy and others you don't, an agent will need to like your kind of writing before they take you on.

When you write your letter of approach, let the agent know whether you are writing to a number of agents at the same time and whether you already have interest from a publisher.

If an agent feels that they may be able to take you on, set up a meeting. In any relationship, no matter how suitable someone might seem on paper, they may not appeal in person. You will be working closely with your agent, and if there is no mutual respect and liking it will be difficult for you to work together. The ideal agent will share your appreciation of your subject and enjoy being part of the process of introducing it to readers.

Alternatives

If, for whatever reason, you don't sell your books through an agent, it is worth considering joining the Society of Authors.[3] This is an independent organisation with around 7500 members which offers individual advice on publishing matters. It keeps up to date with publishing terms and the marketplace, and also campaigns for better publishing and book-selling conditions. The Writers' Guild is a trade union for professional writers and negotiates minimum terms agreements.[4] Both organisations work on an annual subscription basis.

References

1 Turner B. *The Writer's Handbook 2006*. London: Pan; 2005.
2 Pratchett T. *Writers' and Artists' Yearbook 2006*. London: A & C Black; 2005.
3 The Society of Authors; www.societyofauthors.net/
4 The Writers' Guild; www.writersguild.org.uk/

Chapter 7

Writing the book

Gill Wakley

Making time

One of the commonest questions people ask authors is 'How do you find the time?' Like anything else, if you want to do it, you will find the time. If you have not written before, look at Chapter 1, where we suggest how long it takes to write. You may be quicker (we doubt it!) or slower, but it is a guide when you are making your plans. In Chapter 4, you looked at how to make a Gantt chart to organise the various deadlines that you have to meet. This tells you roughly how much time you will need to set aside each week over how long a period.

Speed up to spend less time

Train yourself to write fast. Resist the temptation to make corrections as you go along. Instead, keep the thoughts in your mind and conduct them through your fingers on to the screen or paper. You will have to go through it again anyway, so why interrupt the flow of ideas by correcting your spelling, punctuation or order of words?

Become familiar with your word-processing package, if necessary going on a course before you start. Use its facilities to make your task easier. Set up a template for your writing so that you can easily click on the heading you want (*see* Box 7.1) or design the text to correspond with how you want it set out.

Box 7.1 Using 'Word' to select your headings

The word-processing package will have certain 'styles' set up. If you prefer them to have a different font (letter) size, spacing or emphasis, you can modify them. It helps to have a sequence of headings. For example:

Chapter heading (Arial 16 pt size in bold)
Section heading (Times New Roman 14 pt in bold)
Subheading (Times New Roman 12 pt in bold)

With your text in Normal or Body text (Times New Roman 12 pt line spacing double)

If you know how to do simple formatting tasks, like setting up bulleted or numbered lists and making boxes and tables, your work can be set out the way you would like it to look as you go along. If you have to ask a secretary to do this, you build in a delay.

If you are not already a fast typist, learn. You might want to use a voice-recognition software package such as *Dragon Naturally Speaking* or *IBM Via Voice*. Cheaper packages tend to have lower rates of word recognition. You may be tempted by a dictation package if you are a 'hunt-and-peck' typist, but your typing speed will have improved tremendously by the time you have finished writing a book! Voice recognition is certainly useful if you have any hand pain. Learn to use it and train it in advance so that it recognises your voice instructions. If you are already a speedy typist then it will probably not save time, as the error rate and subsequent corrections are irritating. You have to remember not to swear, say 'er' or 'um', or make other extraneous noises that the voice-recognition software will try to turn into words. Your environment must be relatively quiet as well. If there are other people talking, other noises going on in the background (the builders drilling or hammering, or a lorry rattling by) you will acquire many words you did not intend.

Fitting in the writing

Something in your life will have to go in order to free up the time to write. Take a look at all the projects and activities you are currently working on, not just other writing but in your whole life. Try to eliminate a few things. Analyse your days and work out exactly where the time is going, if necessary writing down what you are doing every half hour of the day for a short while. Cut back on some of the less important tasks. Ration your time spent watching television or reading fiction. Spend less time on the Internet and be ruthless about weeding out your emails. Find someone else to do the decorating or the gardening that you were intending to do. Go out less often. Decide that your work will not spill over into time at home and control it. Make some sacrifices – use your holiday, your early mornings, your evenings or your weekends, especially if you can find occasions when you could use spare time as effectively as Ruth does in Box 7.2.

Box 7.2 Using time for writing that might otherwise be frittered away

Ruth is quite often away overnight with her work, occasionally for two or three nights at a time. She often writes a chapter for a book while away from home, writing 500–1000 words in one- or two-hour bursts. She writes on the train as she travels to and from the venue. She also writes while at the venue, before the meeting starts in the morning, or between the end of the day's conference (e.g. 5.30 p.m.) and dinner (e.g. 7.30 p.m.), and later in the evening when dinner is over (e.g. 10.00 p.m.), instead of going to the bar. In this way she can achieve the right balance for her of working, socialising and quiet activity.

Decide that your writing is worth it, but keep a sense of proportion in all of this. If you cut yourself off from **all** other people and other activities, your writing may become laboured and lacking in sparkle. You may lose friends, partners and other relationships and miss some fun if you shut yourself off too effectively.

Avoiding distractions

Use an answerphone when you are writing so that you are not tempted to pick up the telephone when it rings. Work away from other distractions such as letters, bills, and that interesting article you were going to read on a non-related subject. If you write at home and people call, make it clear that you are working. Be organised so that you can just get on with the writing, rather than wasting time looking for that paper you were going to reference, or the file you thought you had saved in this folder.

Set aside a dedicated session for writing

You may prefer to get your chores of paying bills, making a meal and answering your emails out of the way first, or you may be quite happy to ignore them until later. If you worry about the chores and the worry distracts you, do them now. If you are creative in the early morning, can you organise your day to write then? If your brain is not in gear until midday, and you are at your best in the evening, schedule your writing to fit in then. Ensure that most days include a session of writing. If you are enthused by your writing and have the capacity, the session should be several hours long. If you have very short periods available, they are best reserved for revisions and thinking about the next section of writing. You may be happy to sit still and write for several hours at a time, but some people find that a disciplined routine of stopping for thought and a stretch works well (*see* Box 7.3) for keeping them focused on what needs to be done.

Box 7.3

Ruth gets up and wanders into the kitchen, thinking about what she is about to write as she makes a cup of weak coffee. Sometimes that prompts her to look for other resources while she drinks her coffee, or she will take her coffee back to the computer.

 Gill sets a kitchen timer. When it goes off, she gets up and uses an exercise machine in the study, or walks up and down the stairs for five minutes, while continuing to think about what she is writing.

You may have the opportunity to use a holiday interval or a work-free time to write for several days or weeks sequentially. If you are away from home, make sure that you have everything you need with you – you will need all your resources as well as the laptop in your country cottage or hotel. Take your writing with you whenever you can, as Ruth does in Box 7.2. You can use those times when you are waiting for something, or travelling on a train, or having an unanticipated break because the person you were expecting has not turned up.

Postponing the task

Writing is not for everyone. If you keep trying, and failing, to make time to write, then it may not be for you. You may want to write, but if the desire is not enough to keep you from doing what you regard as more interesting or pressing activities, then perhaps writing is not for you at this moment. When it is important enough for you to make the sacrifices, you will be able to make them. Until then, adjust to the fact that writing is something you would like to do, but not necessarily enough to be a writer of a book that requires a sustained effort. Please give this book to someone else, as reading it will not make you into a writer. Only the hard work of sitting down and writing something that someone else will read makes you a writer. So **start now**.

Overcoming writer's block

It is common for inexperienced writers to fear that they will stare at a blank screen wondering where to start. You should have some ideas in your mind before you start. You cannot start writing without doing some preliminary work or reflection. After you have collected your resources, you need to spend time thinking about how you will order the material and write about it. Have a look at the section on 'Making your writing plan' later in this chapter.

If you are writing about a subject that is not very interesting, try and imagine yourself being in the shoes of someone who needs this information. Craft your words into a journey of discovery for them as you lead them towards the information that they need. Write as though the reader is a student who knows very little, or one who disputes everything that you say.

If you find yourself writing a sentence or a paragraph, then revising it, then deleting it and writing something else, take a break. Put your mind in gear and think about what it is you need to say before trying again. If it is just that you cannot think how to put your idea on the screen or on paper, try writing 'what I mean to say is something about . . .' and writing in what it is you need to write about. You can craft it into brilliant sentences later. Alternatively, take a short break and then tackle another part of your writing, while the section you have struggled over mulls away at the back of your mind. Sometimes you need a longer break away from it. Carrying out some physical activity that occupies your body while allowing your brain to go on sorting things out is often effective. A walk, a workout, cooking, painting – anything that does not require too much brain work.

You do not need to start at the beginning of any writing. A first chapter, or an introduction, is often best written, or augmented, after the rest of the book when you know the contents. You do not need to start at the beginning of a chapter either. If you are using case studies and you find these interesting and stimulating to write, start there. Then draft out what information you require to wrap around the case studies to make them meaningful. Or the other way round – if you have difficulty thinking of case scenarios, write the text and find what specific points you need to illustrate.

Talking it over with someone else may help you to understand how you are going to put this down on paper. If you have a co-author, they are ideal. If not, talk to someone who knows a little about the subject, to bounce around ideas.

Whether face to face, over the telephone, or by email, just start to formulate your ideas. If there is no one you can ask, verbalise your ideas and record them on a tape recorder, or make a mind map (*see* page 70).

If you are stuck for ideas, try pretending that you are someone else – someone you know who lectures on this subject, or a fictional character who might be writing this book instead of yourself. Think how they might approach the section that is blocking you.

A buddy, coach or co-author can help to keep you on track, encourage and support you. If you have a blank about what else you need to put into a section or chapter, leave a space, put in a row of asterisks or a plea for some other material, and give them what you have written so far. Or send them a plaintive email or make a phone call.

Making your writing plan

If you already have a book to write, look back at your book proposal and Gantt chart (*see* Chapters 3 and 4), as these give you the framework for your plan. The detail will help you to know what you are going to write and by when. If you are still formulating your ideas, your plan will help you with the book proposal as well. Think of it as a journey that needs a map or a guide to make sure that you have everything you need (although you can acquire some extra things on the way), know where you are going and how to get there, who will help you on the way, and how you will know when you are there. Figure 7.1 shows your plan in outline. You may share some of these tasks if you are writing with co-authors.

Define the purpose of your book

Look at Chapter 2 for suggestions about the type of book that you might write. Decide:

- why you are writing
- what to include
- what to leave out.

Try recording your purpose in one or two sentences, as in the examples shown in Box 7.4.

Box 7.4 Two examples of statements of the purpose of a book

1 The book will help doctors, nurses and allied health professionals to undertake clinical audit of any part of their clinical practice, but especially with regard to chronic disease management, a current priority for the NHS.
2 This book will be a practical resource to help the general practice team and the primary care organisation to undertake chronic disease management according to best practice, based on problem-based learning.

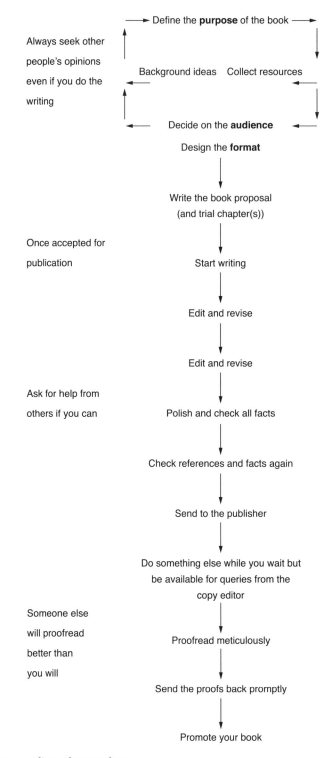

Figure 7.1 An outline of your plan.

The ideas and the resources

You may have ideas at any time. Make sure that you have a notebook, Post-it notes, a notepad, a tape recorder or a personal organiser available both day and night in your bag, your car or by your bed, to record that sudden flash of insight, or that plan, or that significant thought.

You will have been collecting material for your book for months. When you are ready to make your plan, put the material you have gathered into some kind of order. Some of it will consist of paper articles, cuttings and books, while other items will be online websites or downloaded material. If you are working with someone else, their ideas and resources will add to yours and you may need a face-to-face meeting with them to organise their material into your outline. You might want to use the technique of mind mapping to tease out all the various connections (*see* Figure 7.2). A mind map consists of the central concept (i.e. a book on a particular subject) with lines connecting this to all the other facets that make up the book. You will have many more than are shown in this example. Then you can sort them into groups by using highlighter pens, different shapes of boxes, or any other visual technique that you prefer.

An outline works in a similar way, but you group the ideas that you have written on a piece of paper under the main headings, and then divide those main headings into sections as in the listed chapters in the book proposal in Chapter 4. Always leave it for a day or two if you can, and then return to it with a fresh eye to add or delete points and issues.

Decide on your audience

Who are your potential readers? Look at Chapter 2 for some examples. They may be:

- colleagues and others in the same field as yourself
- administrators, local or national government
- a narrow range of health workers
- a broad range of health and/or social workers
- the general public
- a section of the general public with a special interest.

The readership shapes the range of what you include and leave out in your book outline. Go back and look at the contents list to consider whether you need to modify the target audience or the purpose of the book.

Design the format

The layout of your book should be something similar to the following:

- a working title – the publisher may suggest another that is more likely to sell the book
- a contents list – much the same as your chapter outline for your book proposal
- a foreword – preferably written by someone the readers have heard of, to recommend the book

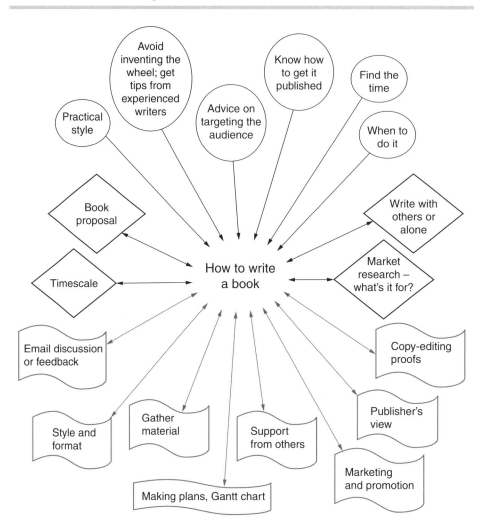

Figure 7.2 Mind map for a book.

- a preface – in which you explain why you have written the book (not essential)
- an introduction – often Chapter 1, but it can be a stand-alone chapter to explain the relevance or context of the book or how to use it
- several chapters to explain in detail what you are writing about
- a summary at the end with recommendations, depending on the type of book
- appendices for material that your readers will find easier to look at here than in another reference book or journal, or unpublished material (e.g. a questionnaire or recording form).

The format and layout of the book are important. You will not have total responsibility for these. The publisher will have to take decisions about matters such as how much white space (i.e. paper with nothing written on it) is allowed around the text, whether colour is permitted, and whether and how many illustrations of what type can be included, as all of these increase costs. Look at

Chapter 8 for guidance on how style can help people to find their way in a book and help to make your arguments or points clearer.

Edit and revise

While writing your chapters you will often find gaps or ideas that prompt you to look for other resources and information. Your outline is not sacrosanct – revise it as you go along, if necessary by consultation with your co-authors or, if a major change is envisaged, with your publisher. The context may have changed in a way that you could not have predicted (e.g. as a result of some natural disaster or new legislation).

Once you have drafted your chapters, the hard work begins. Use the advice in Chapter 8 on style to look critically at your writing, preferably after a short gap of time. Remove superfluous words, and correct spelling and grammar. Look at your outline again. Have you included everything? If you have added material that was not in the outline and it is not relevant, delete it. Put it aside again before repeating the process, or if you have a co-author ask them to do so. Beware of muddling up the various versions that you now have. Have a system of saving them, perhaps with the date or the version number in the footer, so that you know which is the latest and best version. Not everyone saves previous versions, but you may decide to leave out something that you or your adviser later think should be included after all. Back up any versions that you have worked hard to revise, and keep the copy in a safe place. It can be devastating to lose your last hour's work if you have an IT glitch, but to lose your draft book will seem an even more personal loss.

Polishing

Get help. Ask your friends, your colleagues, your co-author, a coach, a mentor – almost anyone you trust – to read your draft and give you feedback. They will spot errors, do the preliminary proofreading, make suggestions and usually give you praise for the good bits. You can send different chapters to different people according to their special interests – it is a lot to ask someone to read a whole book and give you feedback.

Look at your book critically yourself. Eliminate any repetition unless it is there for a specific purpose. Check that you have not left any gaps. Explain any technical terms and ensure that all abbreviations are written out in full at least the first time they are used. Read it aloud. How does it sound? Can you improve the writing still further? Check all your facts, especially if you have used drug dosages or any directions, and confirm that your references are accurate and properly set out (*see* Chapter 8).

Send the manuscript to the publisher

Check that you know how the publisher wants the manuscript to be presented. Common requirements are for double spacing, good margins, one or two paper copies and a text file in a commonly used word-processing package such as Word. You can often send the text file as an attachment by email, although some publishers prefer a floppy disk or CD to be posted with the paper copy.

Be available for the copy editor

The wait that ensues is painful. The editor at the publishers will have several other books on the go. The only reason for prioritising your book would be an agreement with the publisher to fast-track it because of marketing considerations.

The editor and copy editor will have queries. Answer these as quickly as possible, usually within a few days. If you have to consult other people (e.g. another writer or a source), give them a deadline for response. You will realise from the queries how easy it is for readers to misunderstand what you had thought you had made completely clear.

Proofreading

Although you have responsibility for proofreading, someone else reading the book for the first time, or from a different perspective, will find more and different errors compared with yourself. Proofreading is boring – each word must be looked at, not just the sense of what is written. Some people read it forwards and backwards – the backwards reading helping them to focus on separate words. Others read aloud or use a ruler or pen to prevent the eye from skipping over faults or racing ahead. You might find the following tips helpful.

- You need to check for spelling, grammar and punctuation. Ensure that you know the rules for apostrophes.[1]
- Break it up into small sections – do not try to read the whole book in one go.
- Avoid distractions. Ruth proofreads on the train where she knows she will not be interrupted. Gill uses a coloured pen to follow the words so that she knows exactly where she is on the page.
- Look separately at the headings. Are they the right ones for this chapter or section? Spot any variations in heading size or changes in bullet points or style.
- If you are proofreading before sending the book off, avoid relying on proofreading on screen. Your eyes are more used to reading words on paper, and errors that you might gloss over on screen will jump out at you on paper.
- Ask for help. You are familiar with what has been written and will tend to skip over parts that you spent time revising. Other people will spot different mistakes. Ruth and Gill always find that each notices different errors, as well as a lot of the same ones. The copy editor **always** discovers some errors that we have missed.

Send the proofs back as promptly as possible. You will usually have a deadline, and time is short.

Book promotion

It is your book, and you will have the greatest impetus to promote it. Take one of your free-to-author copies with you everywhere, as you will often be able to display it or mention it. If someone can hold it and flick through it, they are more likely to remember it. Publishers usually produce fliers – glossy printed single sheets with details of your book, sometimes with related titles listed as well. You may be able to negotiate that a flier could be inserted in every folder at a relevant conference, or leave a supply for people to pick up. Some conferences have bookstalls, in which case mention to the organiser that your book should be available for the bookstall to sell. Mention your book in talks and workshops and in conversation. If you are shy, fewer people will buy your book and all that work will be wasted. Turn to Chapter 10 for information about the publisher's perspective on and insights into promoting a book.

Reference

1 Truss L. *Eats, Shoots and Leaves: the zero tolerance approach towards punctuation.* London: Profile Books Ltd; 2003.

Chapter 8

Style

Gill Wakley

Presenting your work well helps to convince publishers that you can write and will be read. Writing well requires thought and care, but will increase your readership.

Design and layout

Spend time in bookshops watching people inspecting non-fiction books. They pick them up, often because of the cover, but may be seen searching for titles on a subject they need. They usually flick through the book, looking at the general shape and layout, before looking at the contents list or reading some of the content. Dense text without anything to break it up looks boring and hard work to a reader. Too much white space in a workbook may make them decide that they can supply their own paper for writing at less cost. Time spent on the appearance of a book is not wasted. As an author, you do have a major influence on the way that the publisher designs the final imprint of the book, building on your preferred format. However, your suggested design must fit with the publisher's usual in-house layout.

While you are in the bookshop, look at the books themselves. Judge which kind of layout would best suit the category of book that you are writing. The publisher will have the best knowledge for many of the decisions that need to be made – bindings, covers, print size, etc. – but you should decide on the best layout and design for your text. Once you have decided on how it should look, keep to a uniform layout for all the chapters, except perhaps the introduction or first chapter. This is particularly important in a multi-author book. Box 8.1 shows the type of leadership you need to give other co-authors. Email your template to all the authors, or write a chapter and email that as the guide for other people's writing.

Box 8.1

Gill was asked to write a chapter for a multi-author book. She was not given any guidance on how to set out the chapter, but from her previous experience and knowledge of the publications from that source, she drew up her own layout. She wrote quicker than anyone else, and the chapter arrived back with the editors of the book. They were pleased not to have to draw up a specification for the layout, and circulated the chapter to demonstrate to other contributors how their chapters should be set out.

Activity boxes

If you are writing a workbook, you might want to give the reader exercises to do and record in the book, so plan how you will fit this into the text, as shown in Box 8.2. Do you place them at the end of each chapter or in the break between sections in a chapter?

Box 8.2 Example of an activity for the reader, to break up the text

Activity 2 To rate communication techniques

Work in trios, one acting as instructor, one as learner and one as observer. Try out different techniques, the observer recording and writing comments before you all discuss what happened at the end of the 10-minute session.

	Helps	Hinders	Comments
Eye contact			
Hand movements			
How you sit or stand			
How close you are			
Etc.			

The activity can be in the form of a blank box with just a heading, a series of tick boxes to complete, or a series of questions to answer. You might use a particular icon to flag successive activities and identify what level or type of activity or information is being given at that point, as we did in *Improving Sexual Health Advice*.[1] You can target particular readers and make your book stand out as different from its competitors (*see* Box 8.3).

Box 8.3 Example from the publisher's catalogue

The Problem-Based Learning Workbook

Key Clinical Scenarios for Medical Undergraduates

T M French and T D Wardle

The scenarios in this unique workbook have been written by consultants, registrars, house officers and medical students, to demonstrate the range of issues with which students at all levels will have to become familiar in order to evolve into competent medical practitioners. Each scenario is followed by questions with an extensive range of sensible answers. It is extensively illustrated and lists a full range of further reading and Web-based resources.

2006 ● Paperback 272 pages ● Radcliffe Publishing
ISBN 1 85775 736 X

Match the layout to the book

A synopsis or brief notes on a subject will have a heading followed by the text in short sections, often arranged by subject, alphabetically (an A to Z of . . .), chronologically (Treating disease x from development to conclusion) or by likelihood of occurrence (Differential diagnosis of . . .).

A reference resource inevitably contains a lot of tables. Ensure that the reader can read them, and break them up into shorter, less complex tables whenever possible.

A narrative account or historical book will have longer sections of text divided up into time sections or aspects of the account. The divisions are by chapter headings or a double space before a subsequent section of a chapter, rather than by headings and subheadings.

A textbook or an information book needs an imaginative layout to give it shape and a distinctive character with case studies, titles, subtitles and sections. Use lists and quotes to break up the text into shorter sections.

Box 8.4 An example of a layout

In the series entitled *Demonstrating Your Competence*,[2] Ruth and Gill discussed at length how the layout should look.

They decided on an introductory first chapter that explained the background and how to use the book. The rest of the chapters were divided into a first section that laid out the bare bones of the subject under discussion with references to more information, followed by three practical examples of how you might go about demonstrating your competence in that subject. The practical examples were based on a case study in a box, followed by numbered stages to work through. The stages were based on a repeated logo of an evidence cycle placed at the beginning of each example.

As in this book, they used boxes for examples and further information, bulleted or numbered lists with a consistent format, and headings for sections of information, with subheadings where the information needed further division.

Anecdotes to break up the text must obviously be completely relevant to the topic. Be cautious, as unless the anecdote rings true with readers and they can identify with the subject or people, it may be counter-productive. If it makes the reader think 'What a stupid person', 'I would never do that' or alternatively 'This person is not practising in the same world as me', you have antagonised them and lost their attention.

Before and after the main text

Before the book proper comes the material known as the front matter (*see* Box 8.5).

Box 8.5 Front matter

The parts of a book that appear before the actual text are referred to as the front matter. They include the following:
- pages which the publisher will produce, containing information about them
- a title page containing the draft title and authors' names
- a page for copyright notification
- a dedication or acknowledgements, if any
- table of contents
- foreword
- preface
- list of contributors or authors, with a brief outline (*see* below)
- list of abbreviations, acronyms or glossary.

These pages are not included in the arabic-numeral pagination, but are usually given small roman numerals.

The material at the end of the book (end matter) includes the index, usually arranged by the publishers (for which we are very grateful), and any appendices.

Listing co-authors or contributors

Editors and co-authors often have a brief CV in the front matter. You need to decide on the style for these. You may want to use first names, or be formal and state titles and qualifications. The CV should give some indication of an author's or co-author's authority to be writing the book or chapter. Make them fairly short – around 100 words is enough to make the point that you are an experienced person in this field and able to tell readers what they should do from an expert standpoint! Editors and co-authors should decide on the order of their names on the title page, usually on the basis of how much work each of them did. Sometimes you will want to put the best-known name first because that author in lead position is more likely to encourage people to buy and read the book. Less commonly there will be political, financial or hierarchical reasons for the order of names.

Contributors to edited books are usually paid per contribution (e.g. a chapter) rather than receiving royalties. The fee may, of course, be in kind – free books, or just the glory (*see* Chapter 3). The editor or editors are responsible for liaising with contributors, correcting their copy and fielding the copy editor's queries. You can include a short CV for each contributor. This may be similar to that for the editors or kept very short, consisting only of their name, qualifications and place of work. Decide on the format and insist on its use for everyone. If a contributor who was asked for a CV of around 50 words writes 250 words of biographical detail, you or a co-editor must reduce it down to match the rest. Ask for the CV well ahead of the time when you need it, as contributors frequently lose interest in your project once their own chapter has been finalised.

Remember to let the publisher's editor know which writers will need copies of the proofs and who is the main author or editor for correspondence.

People who have helped in a minor way, by reading through and commenting, proofreading, giving you a quote or a paragraph, or putting up with your obsessive and antisocial behaviour while undertaking the project, are usually thanked in the acknowledgments section.

Organising paragraphs

A paragraph is a group of sentences (or just one sentence) related to a particular topic or idea, and it makes one main point. The topic sentence (usually the first sentence) states this central idea, and the rest of the sentences develop it using the following:

- examples to illustrate it (like the boxes in this chapter)
- lists (like this one)
- classifying or defining terms (*see* Box 8.6)
- comparing and contrasting (look at the 'pros and cons' Boxes in Chapter 3).

Box 8.6[2] Classifying and defining terms

Risk factors for osteoporosis	Types of osteoporosis
	Primary
- Female gender	- Type 1 (postmenopausal)
- Elderly	- Type 2 (age-related bone loss)
- Early menopause	- Idiopathic (onset before 50 years of age)
- Smoking	
- High alcohol intake	**Secondary**
- Physical inactivity	- Endocrine (thyrotoxicosis, primary hyperparathyroidism, Cushing's syndrome, hypogonadism due to anorexia nervosa or excessive exercise)
- Thin body type	
- Heredity	
- Other causes of secondary osteoporosis (*see* next column)	- Gastrointestinal (malabsorption due to coeliac disease, partial gastrectomy, liver disease)
	- Rheumatological (rheumatoid arthritis, ankylosing spondylitis)
	- Malignancy (multiple myeloma, metastases)
	- Corticosteroids

Once you have individual paragraphs organised logically, the next step is to organise all the paragraphs in a coherent way to make things easy for your readers.

- **Chronologically** – start with what happened first (or last) and work through each event in the order in which it occurred.

- **Spatially** – around specific places or areas (e.g. you might group them by what happens in England, Scotland, Wales and Northern Ireland, or by different groups of patients).
- **Readership** – you might ask people to rate their own learning needs and read different sections accordingly, as in *Improving Sexual Health Advice*.[1] You could group your paragraphs according to occupation or area of responsibility.
- **Comparison or contrast** – especially if you are putting forward diverse points of view or one for which there is no clear solution. This also lends itself to rating items in order of importance (e.g. writing about common before rare causes of illness), or less charged emotional aspects to more highly charged ones (e.g. when talking about sexual abuse or genital mutilation).
- **Order of difficulty** – present the more easily understood parts first, before the complicated sections.
- **Building an argument** – a device, often used in fiction, that can add suspense and interest to presenting your conclusion with a final flourish.

Headings

Apart from breaking up the text and guiding your reader towards what it is you are talking about next, headings are used to collect information for the contents list. Most copy editors use the main chapter heading (often known as a level 1 heading), the section heading (level 2 heading) and the subheading (level 3 heading) to identify what is important. You may have your chapter headings in point (type) size 16 at level 1, your section headings in point size 14 at level 2 and your subheadings in point size 13 at level 3. Other subsidiary headings that are not important enough to be listed in the contents (e.g. headings in example boxes) can be at level 4 or below, perhaps in point size 12. Put the heading levels 1, 2 and 3 for your headings into your template for ease and convenience.

Text formatting

Fonts

Word processing offers too many fonts (typefaces). Resist the temptation to use more than one or two. The publisher will use another font in any case. Type size is measured in points. Write in at least point size 12, as typesetters will reduce size 10 (which you might have used for text in a box or table) down to minute letters that are difficult to read. If you are writing for the visually handicapped, the Royal National Institute for the Blind recommends a mimimum of point size 14, but you will have to negotiate larger print with your publisher.

Avoid using capital letters for emphasis unless you REALLY WANT TO SHOUT. **Bold is better for emphasis** and easier to read. Reserve underlining for website links. Use italics for the titles of books (and names of ships, operas, plays and films), proper Latin names of plants, animals and bacteria, etc. You might use italics in a list to separate out categories, or for a quotation. Overuse of italics or any font variation makes the text difficult to read.

Line length affects the speed of reading. Very long sentences have to be read several times, and very short sentences can be jerky if used frequently. Keep the interest of the reader with varying lengths of sentence, and avoid very long sentences with many subsidiary clauses.

Alignment

Decide on your preferred alignment and keep to it. If you indent the first line of your paragraphs, justify the text (both edges aligned), range the text to the left (with a ragged edge to the right) or centre it, keep to this throughout. Text ranged to the left is easier to read, as justified text varies the spaces between words.

Quotes

A quote should be clearly **not** part of your text. Again, decide on your book style. It is easier to differentiate a quote if it is inset, boxed, or set in a margin or in a different font. Always reference the quote.

Hyphenation

Avoid using hyphens to divide a word at the end of a line. Use the word-processing package to automatically wrap your text so that only whole words appear. Normal hyphens are used in compound words to connect words (e.g. cost-benefit analysis, pre- and postnatal period). There seem to be fashions in publishing for standard grammar such as the use of hyphens – your publisher will probably have a guide for their copy editors that you could look at. Take care to standardise such words as 'self-care' or 'self care' from the beginning. For interest, you may like to know that an 'en rule' is the width of a letter 'n' and is set without any spaces when used in number ranges (e.g. 8–16 years). Use Ctrl + – on the numerical keyboard to insert it. An 'em rule' is the width of a letter 'm' (twice the width of an en rule) and has a space before and after it. Use Alt Ctrl – on the numerical keyboard to insert it. Unless you are self-publishing, these fine points will be sorted out during typesetting, but check the proofs.

Lists

If you have a long sentence with many commas between items, think about turning it into a list. Decide on, and use throughout, the same type of bulleted or numbered lists, unless you want to make the point that a particular list is different. You can use dashes, arrows and a multitude of devices, with outline lists where there is another list under that bullet or numbered point:

1. this point is first, leading on to
    1.1. this one next
        1.1.1 and then another subsidiary point here.

If you have a long list, try to break it up into more than one list, or a sentence (with not more than three items) and a list.

Note that the full stop is usually placed at the end of the list. If you start each item of the list with a capital letter, it is customary to place a full stop at the end if it is a sentence, but not if it is a single word or a short phrase. If the list is a continuation of a sentence that introduced the list, use a lower-case letter at the beginning of each item and a full stop at the end of the list. Whatever you decide, keep to it throughout, and check that it is consistent when you proofread your manuscript.

Quotation marks and brackets

Take a decision to use single quotation marks unless the quote is clearly part of a conversation (the convention in the UK). Alternatively, you may decide to always use double or single quotation marks, even for conversations. Then keep to what you have decided on throughout the book. Reserve the use of the more elaborate types of brackets – other than simple curved parentheses – for specific purposes (e.g. curly brackets for equations, square brackets for the date you accessed a website reference).

Spelling, abbreviations and acronyms

In non-fiction writing, you use technical words, people's names, obscure Latin names, and many words that are simply not in the spellchecker of the average word-processing package. Trade names for pharmaceuticals and devices start with an upper-case letter, whereas generic names start with a lower-case letter. Examples are shown in Box 8.7.

Box 8.7

1 'We stocked generic aciclovir and the once daily preparation Famvir.'
2 'Patients were offered a choice between a copper intrauterine device (Cu IUD) and Mirena©, a progesterone-bearing intrauterine system (IUS).'
3 'He showed signs of impetigo, caused by *Staphylococcus aureus.*'
4 'She suffered from candida, caused by *Candida albicans.*'

Note: © = copyright and can be inserted using Alt + 0169 using the numerical keyboard with the numbers lock on.

Check and check again that all spellings, abbreviations and acronyms are correct, and then check them again when you proofread. Remember that there are differences in spelling between countries – we 'practise' medicine in the UK whereas we 'practice' medicine in the USA. Book reviewers and readers just love to catch you out!

There are standard abbreviations – e.g., etc., i.e. and others – that need not be explained. If you are unsure of the conventions for these, use a reference source.[3] If your book has a large number of technical words and abbreviations, compile a glossary, which is conventionally placed at the end of the front matter (*see* Box 8.5) in the book, before the first page of the main text. Acronyms, which are a form of abbreviation, must also be explained. One person's DOA (dead on arrival in Accident and Emergency) is another's DOA (date of admission on the ward). Pelvic inflammatory disease and prolapsed intervertebral disc (PID) are less likely to be confused because of the context. CHD is often coronary heart disease, but could be County Health Director. If you have an uncommon acronym, you can check it by referring to any of several Internet resources.[4] Avoid starting a sentence with an acronym. A piece of text that is full of acronyms is difficult to read, especially if they are unfamiliar to the reader and he or she has to repeatedly refer to the glossary or, worse, to wherever the acronym was first used in the book (*see* Box 8.8).

Box 8.8 Too many acronyms

The importance of local and national agencies such as the RCP, ASH and the BMA, as well as HEAs with HAs, LAs and FSHAs, in taking the lead in the promotion of health has been clearly illustrated in the case of cigarette smoking and more recently to prevent the spread of HIV/AIDS.

Use internationally accepted signs and symbols for units. If you are unfamiliar with the ones you will be using (e.g. units used in spirometry), look them up.[5]

Remember to check for words that are not picked up by a spellchecker. For example, 'there' and 'their', 'two', 'too' and 'to', and 'buy' and 'by' may be confused.

Tables

The publisher may have requirements for these, so check whether this is the case. For example, one publisher includes the following in their requirements:

> Tables are structured using horizontal lines above and below the column headings and a line beneath the columns. If necessary for clarity, further lines, both horizontal and vertical, may be inserted.

In general, the simpler the tables and figures, the easier they are to read. Tables should have at least two columns and two rows. Otherwise you can incorporate the material in the text as a list or in a box. Use a large enough font size and not too much information. Consider using symbols (*see* Box 8.9) or superscript letters (lower case a, b, c, etc.) to denote what items mean, and putting the explanation of the symbols or letters at the bottom (or top) of the table. This avoids cluttering up the numbers in the table. List your abbreviations (yes, you will almost certainly have them) at the bottom of the table as well.

Box 8.9 Example of use of symbols and abbreviations

Cardiovascular risk factors in people with diabetes

	Low	*Borderline*	*High*
BP	<130/80*	140/80–150/90**	>150/90§
Sm	No	Ex-smoker	Current smoker
BMI	>25	26–30	>30
Etc.			

BP = blood pressure (mmHg), Sm = smoking status, BMI = body mass index (kg/m^2).
* Advice varies between guidelines, and lower readings may be advised.
** Treatment may be advised at any of these levels by different guidelines.
§ Treatment is always advised.

If you are writing for the non-technical reader, you must explain what the numbers mean. For instance, in the example above explain that the upper figure is the systolic blood pressure and the lower one is diastolic blood pressure, and how these numbers are obtained.

If you are using equations, simple ones can be entered as text. Complicated ones are better pasted in as a text object from the original file. With the exception of mathematicians and health economists, readers tend to regard equations as a turn-off and put the book back on the shelf.

Use a legend (a title) to explain each figure. Some publishers will prefer this to be inserted under the figure, rather than above it. It is often preferable to draw your figure in another file and paste it in, or to indicate its position in the text, so that it is entire and does not become muddled up in the text. You can use a figure created in other software packages such as a PowerPoint presentation. You must obtain permission if the figure was originally someone else's work (*see* below).

Remember to check that your boxes, tables and figures are numbered consecutively and that your numbering system is consistent. Refer to boxes, tables and figures in the text by their number without indicating their position relative to that reference (for example, *see* Box 9.1 below). The publisher may alter the positioning of the box, table or figure in the midst of your text to fit in with the page layout, or so that it does not start at the bottom of one page and end halfway down another.

References

Decide whether you will put references at the end of each chapter, at the end of the book or, if there are only a few, as footnotes on the pages where they are cited. Find out what system the publisher uses. Two main systems exist in the UK for medical and bioscience publishing – the Vancouver and the Harvard systems.[6] The Vancouver system is known as the author-number system, and the Harvard as the author-date system. We have used the Vancouver system in this book. A superscript number, or a number in brackets, goes unobtrusively after the words you wish to reference, and the reference at the end of the chapter lists them in **numerical order**, making them easy to find. Look up how to set out the entries for the references, as specific rules apply (e.g. Wakley G. Questionnaires: paradigms and pitfalls. *J Fam Plann Reprod Health Care* 2005; **31**(3): 222–224).

If you use the Harvard system, insert the author's last name and the date in parentheses (curved brackets) (e.g. (Chambers, 2006)) and list the references in **alphabetical** order at the end. Again, there are specific conventions with regard to how they should be written, whether for a book, an article, a chapter in a book, etc. Look these up and follow them meticulously. If you use a reference bibliography software package such as Reference Manager or Endnote, it will usually insert references for you in the required style.

Many publishers, universities and institutions use variations on the two main styles, so check whether this is the case and, if necessary, set up your bibliography programme to insert them correctly. If you are writing for a publisher in the USA, check to see what is required and consult the detailed system. For example, *The Chicago Manual of Style* illustrates two systems, the author-date system and the documentary note style.[7] Another source, from Dartmouth College,[8] gives the often used American Psychological Association (APA) citation style and the Modern Language Association (MLA) citation style, but also quotes the *Science* citation style, which is a condensed endnote format used by the journal *Science*, as well as the Note style, as recommended by the *MLA Handbook for Writers of Research Papers.* Agree a way of citing personal anecdotes or communications that are not part of a report. Citing a reference can be a real minefield!

Illustrations

Pictures break up the text and make the book look more attractive. They add value in that the visual image can often explain something better and more briefly than a long section of text. A book on skin diseases would be of little value to the reader without photographs. Surgical techniques can be more easily illustrated with a line drawing or a diagram superimposed on a photograph. Cartoons are useful in a book for the more general reader, but might put off someone looking for a serious textbook. Unless you are a professional illustrator, ask the publisher for advice. Line drawings in black and white can be inserted fairly easily using software programmes such as Corel Draw or Adobe Illustrator. Photographs usually have to be in a specific format. If the publisher cannot afford colour reproduction, convert your images to a grey scale and look at them to ensure that they are still clear and show what you want.

Permissions

If an illustration or photograph does not belong to you, you must seek and obtain written permission to publish it. The publisher will want to see the permission. Some publishers have standard forms, or you can copy the form of words from one of these. If you use case studies, either they should be obviously made up, or you must seek permission for publication from the individual concerned and anyone else mentioned. Many authors use composite case histories drawn from a mix of real people's experiences. That way you have a feeling of real life when you read the narrative, but the identities of the several people upon which the case is based are unrecognisable, as only snippets of their details are inserted.

Your own writing

Your style

Think of your reader as you write. You are not trying to impress the reader with fancy words and turgid prose. A book is an exercise in communication. The easier the text is to read, the more understandable information can be transferred from writer to reader. Many writing guides suggest that you write as you speak, but the two techniques are different – as anyone who has transcribed a focus group or conference presentation can testify. In speaking, we use fragments of sentences, repetitions and imprecise words, and we go backwards and forwards between ideas. Reading your written work aloud helps you to achieve comprehension and clarity, but is not the same as recording speech verbatim.

Sentence length

Use short sentences. A good average sentence length is 15 to 20 words.[9] Short sentences convey emphasis. Longer sentences should not contain more than three items of information, so convert a longer sentence into two or more shorter sentences or into a list.

Box 8.10 Long sentences

Example from a book on case studies:

> Absolutely essential parts of a data-gathering plan are the following: definition of case, list of research questions, identification of helpers, data sources, allocation of time, expenses, intended reporting.

Reformat as a list for clarity:

> Essential parts of a data-gathering plan are:
>
> - definition of case
> - list of research questions
> - identification of helpers
> - data sources
> - allocation of time
> - expenses
> - intended reporting.

Or as more than one sentence:

> Essential parts of a data-gathering plan include defining the case, listing the research questions and identifying the helpers. You must also record data sources, the time needed, and how much it will cost. Decide how you will report the case study.

Jargon

Some jargon can be useful – a form of shorthand between people who have similar backgrounds to explain concepts that might otherwise have to be spelt out.

Box 8.11 Jargon

The first recommendation for treatment for obesity is always to advise lifestyle changes.

This is acceptable in a textbook for health professionals. In one for non-specialist readers the jargon should be spelt out by listing exactly what lifestyle changes are advised.

Too much jargon will irritate readers (especially if the jargon is unfamiliar or obscure) and hides the meaning of what you wish to communicate. In the example below, 'the patient's journey' is an expression commonly used by managers in the health service, but is confusing to anyone not familiar with this use of the phrase. Much of the wording here sounds pompous and over-elaborate, obscuring the meaning.

Box 8.12 Jargon to distance any reader who is not part of the 'in-group'

Taken from the National Service Framework (NSF) for Children, Young People and Maternity Services.

Several factors influenced **the selection of exemplar conditions,** for example: large numbers of children and families affected, significant cause of illness and distress, wide variability in standards of practice or service provision and **suitability for highlighting the NSF themes.** Such themes include the importance of responding to the views of children and their parents, involving them in key decisions, providing early identification, diagnosis and intervention, delivering flexible, **child-centred, holistic care. Care is integrated between agencies and over time** and **is sensitive to the individual's changing needs.** It is also acknowledged that not every child with the same condition will **follow the same journey** or have the same type or severity of condition as the one which is illustrated.

This could be rephrased as follows.

Several factors influenced which examples we chose – for instance:

- the large numbers of children and families affected
- severe illness and distress
- wide variability in standards of practice or service provision
- illustrating the themes in the NSF.

The themes in the NSF include the importance of responding to the views of children and their parents and involving them in key decisions. Providing early identification, diagnosis and intervention, and delivering flexible and comprehensive care centred on the child's needs are also important. The agencies involved must cooperate and be flexible with regard to the needs of the child over time. Other children with the same condition may have different needs from those in the examples.

Use active language

Whenever you can, change a passive sentence into an active one, as in Box 8.13. You can usually achieve about 90% active sentences, and you can set your word-processing package to highlight passive sentences for you to convert. The advice recently encountered on an academic website from the USA, to use passive sentences for 'more formality' in academic writing, is old-fashioned, unnecessary and counter-productive. The purpose of a book is not to impress an old and retired teacher but to communicate to readers and help as many people as possible to read your books.

Box 8.13 Converting passive to active text

Women using oral contraception should be advised that some drugs could reduce contraceptive efficacy.

> Change to:
>
> Advise women using oral contraception that some drugs could reduce contraceptive efficacy.

Decide whether you will use the pronouns 'I', 'we' or 'you', and use them consistently throughout the book. The more informal the style, the more likely you are to use pronouns. You will have shorter punchier statements and sentences, as in the example in Box 8.14. Any organisation or group of writers can become 'we', and the reader becomes 'you'.

Box 8.14 Using pronouns

The research protocol was drawn up by the two authors over several months.

Change to:

We drew up the research protocol over several months.

Use everyday words

A passage of text that has to be read with the dictionary to hand is irritating and likely to be put aside until a later date, which never comes. The Plain English website[9] gives a list of commonly encountered words for which a simpler, more easily understood word will do better. Occasional use of a complex or little used word where the meaning is just right for the context may enrich your writing by making it more precise. More commonly it is just showing off, or writing to match the requirements of specialist and little-read journals. Read through the jargon and complex words in Box 8.15 to realise how frustrating such wording can be.

Box 8.15 Examples of jargon and complex words

1 These 'contextual' apologetics are arguably an ethical loophole inherent in current bioethical methodology. However, this convenient appropriation of 'contextual' analysis simply fails to acknowledge the underpinnings of feminist ethical analysis upon which it must stand. A more rigorous analysis of the political, social and economic structures pertaining to the global context of developing countries reveals that the bioethical principles of beneficence and justice fail to be met in this trial design.
2 We show that selection can induce ex ante therapeutic misconception and ex post disappointment among research subjects; and it undermines the rationale of collective equipoise as an ethical basis for clinical trials.

Avoid polysyllabic words, the use of a foreign language when there is an English equivalent, Latin tags, and anything that the target audience will find difficult to read. Most of your readers will be equivalent to readers of serious newspapers. Look at the leader writers and health correspondents and see how they use language. No one has a dictionary on the train or the Tube. If you are writing for the public, look critically at how journalists in the tabloids make their points, using simple words and sentences.

English language rules

The publication of a whole book mainly devoted to the incorrect use of punctuation[10] showed Ruth and Gill that they were not the only ones to be excessively irritated by this. Apostrophes are commonly misused or abused. Their correct usage is described in Box 8.16.

Box 8.16 Examples of the apostrophe's use

Correct usage would be:

   The three **nurses'** uniforms were ruined.

Better to rephrase it as:

   The uniforms of all three nurses were ruined.

Apostrophes after a proper name should be as follows:

   Moses' laws

You might use:

   the laws of Moses

Hers, its, theirs, yours and ours have no apostrophe, but it is **one's** opinion that **someone else's** writing is better. But '**It's** better to be careful than sorry (It is better . . .).'

Matching a phrase to the correct person is essential. In 'grammar language', this states that 'a participial phrase at the beginning of a sentence must refer to the grammatical subject.' Examples make this rule clear (*see* Box 8.17).

Box 8.17 Being clear about what you mean

As a writer of popular books, his computer was quite fast.

The above sentence contains only the computer as the grammatical subject. All becomes clear if you say instead:

As a writer of popular books, he needed to use a fast computer.

While waiting for the kettle to boil, an idea began forming.

How many ideas wait for the kettle to boil? Corrected, this becomes:

*While waiting for the kettle to boil, an idea began forming in **my** head.*

There are many 'rules' of grammar that are frequently broken, like never putting a preposition at the end of a sentence. Not splitting infinitives is another favourite, but we all do it (e.g. the famous 'to boldly go where no man has gone before'). Gill used *Fowler's Modern English Usage* in her last years at school and for some years subsequently. Written 75 years ago (no, she did not buy it then!), it is pedantic and didactic, but was useful and is still available in an updated version.[11] Gill now uses a classic little book called *The Elements of Style* by Strunk and White,[12] also old (first published in 1935, but updated since then). However, Ruth does not refer to such books, relying instead on the regimented training in grammar and tables of her childhood era.

Language is constantly changing, and rules can be broken, but not all the time or the writing becomes difficult to read. This is not the place for a complete run-through of the rules for placing commas, when to use the semi-colon or the colon, or why you should use parentheses or a dash. Buy yourself a little book on the use of the English language and use it as a guide (not a rule book) if you are unsure.

References

1 Wakley G, Cunnion M, Chambers R. *Improving Sexual Health Advice*. Oxford: Radcliffe Medical Press; 2003.
2 Chambers R, Wakley G and various co-authors. *Demonstrating Your Competence* series. Oxford: Radcliffe Publishing; 2004–2006.
3 www.bma.org.uk/ap.nsf/Content/LIBAbbreviations
4 www.lib.umn.edu/libdata/page.phtml?page_id=714#toc17579
5 www.spirxpert.com/indices3.htm
6 www.bma.org.uk/ap.nsf/Content/LIBReferenceStyles
7 www.libs.uga.edu/ref/chicago.html
8 www.dartmouth.edu/~sources/examples/about.html
9 www.plainenglish.co.uk/guides.html
10 Truss L. *Eats, Shoots and Leaves: the zero tolerance approach towards punctuation*. London: Profile Books Ltd; 2003.
11 Allen R. *Pocket Fowler's Modern English Usage*. Oxford: Oxford University Press; 2004.
12 Strunk W, White EB. *The Elements of Style*. 4th ed. New York: Longman; 2000.

Chapter 9

The publisher's side: editorial and production

Gill Nineham

Why publishers ask authors to write

Publishers ask authors to write for a number of different reasons, such as:

- The publisher may have identified a gap in the market that they wish to fill. For example, there may be lots of books for family doctors about caring for older patients, but not one that looks specifically at depression in older people.
- They have a strong publishing programme (or 'list' in publishing jargon) in a particular subject area, and have already produced a number of books in this area. They wish to update the subject, look at it from a different angle, or publish a further text as an introduction, or in more depth, for a different discipline, for a multidisciplinary audience, or for an international audience.
- They have heard some interesting conference presentations that they think deserve to reach a wider audience, and they believe that an editor could develop them into a successful book.
- A series of magazine or journal articles lend themselves to being edited into a book.
- New developments in health or social care policy need to be interpreted for those who will be responsible for or involved in implementing them.
- Changes to the way in which systems are organised result in the need for texts to explain how to cope with those changes.
- New developments in a curriculum require new course texts.
- Research findings result in the need for a book to disseminate them.
- Other publishers have been successful in a particular field, and they believe they can emulate this success.
- They may have published a book that covers a wide topic and they believe that, rather than publish a new edition of the same book, they should break the topic down and publish a series of smaller books looking at different aspects of the topic in greater depth.
- A format has worked in one subject area and they want to replicate it in another.
- They are developing a series on a topic, or for a particular audience, and want additional titles for the series. If this is the case, you are likely to be asked to follow certain guidelines, or a template, when writing your book.
- A successful book exists for academics, and the publisher believes that a more practical handbook for practitioners would be helpful.

- Your previous books have been successful and they believe that the market would welcome another book from you.
- The publisher wishes to expand into new areas or markets and needs a new series of books to start this process.

What does a publisher look for in a book proposal?

Your proposal is your sales tool and needs to grab the publisher's attention immediately. It should be confident and persuasive, and professionally presented with convincing information and accurate detail. A publisher needs to be convinced about the following things.

- There is a need for a book on the topic written in the way that you describe it.
- It is timely. You are going to be able to produce a manuscript and they are going to be able to publish it to reach the market at the most appropriate time. It is not going to go out of date too quickly.
- You are the most appropriate person/people to write it.
- The intended audience needs or will want your book enough to buy it. The publisher will be able to persuade sufficient numbers of people to do so to make it a commercial success.
- There is no other book that already meets the need you have identified.

Introducing your proposal

When a publisher receives a book proposal, it will usually be looked at by a commissioning editor. They will probably receive a large number of proposals, so you need to ensure that their initial look at yours makes them want to read more. A brief introductory paragraph will help them to assess quickly whether your proposal is likely to be of interest. You should include a working title and a brief description of the scope of the book and its content, why it is needed, the audience, style and enough about yourself to demonstrate why you should write it.

Working title

This should obviously reflect the content of the book as closely as possible. If you propose something esoteric, the publisher may suggest a subtitle that spells out exactly what the book is about and whom it is for. The title is sometimes refined or changed when it goes into production.

The content and style of your book

These are discussed in detail in Chapters 2 and 8, respectively. You need to persuade the publisher that you have covered the topic in enough breadth and depth, and that the writing style you propose is appropriate for the book's aims and your audience.

The market for your book

As well as needing to be convinced that there is a market for your book, the publisher will need to feel confident that they can reach that market. Any publisher can produce any book, but effective and efficient marketing, promotion, sales and distribution are key to its success. Furthermore, it is not necessarily enough for the publisher to be a leader in the field of, for example, urology if all their urology books are academic textbooks, and your proposed book is a practical introduction for Foundation Programme doctors. If they don't publish other books for Foundation Programme doctors, it will be costly and inefficient for them to spend time and resources on the marketing and promotion of this one book. This issue is discussed in more depth in Chapter 10.

When defining the market for your book, although it is tempting to indicate a large potential market, be as focused as possible. Saying 'doctors', 'nurses' or 'therapists' is too broad. It is better to focus on a subgroup, such as a particular specialty, nurses at a certain point in their career or working in particular settings or with particular patient groups, or a specific type of therapist or subgroup with a special interest. It may not be necessary to provide numbers of people in these subgroups, as the publisher will probably know this, but if you know them you could include them.

Is there a secondary market for your book? Avoid being overambitious. It is difficult and costly to market widely, and numbers are not all-important. It is better to have a clearly defined group of people who buy books. Is there an international market for your book? Sometimes, particularly in the USA, this will be partly dependent on whether you have international experts contributing chapters.

Identifying competing or complementary books

Unless you are writing about something very new, your book is unlikely to be the only one in its subject area. And if you have chosen to submit your proposal to a publisher that specialises in your area, whether by topic or audience, it is unlikely that it will be the only one published by them. You need to highlight what is new about your book. Perhaps it:

- contains new information or new perspectives on the subject
- covers aspects of the subject that are not covered elsewhere
- is aimed at a different audience – perhaps it is multidisciplinary whereas existing books are aimed at particular professionals
- is written in a different style – there may be a number of monographs or academic textbooks on the subject, but no practical handbooks.

You may be able to put forward other reasons.

The publisher may know about other titles that could be perceived as competition, but it will help if you identify the key ones, especially if you comment on why your book will be different. Demonstrate that you have done your research on what is out there. If it is a popular topic, do not list all the books, but narrow the field to those which are closely related in subject matter, published recently and aimed at a similar readership. You are not required to carry out an exhaustive literature search, or to provide full book reviews, but include information that will support your proposal.

If there are many books published in your area, do not become despondent. This is not necessarily bad news, but demonstrates that publishers believe that there is a good market for them. Moreover, the existing books may be complementary to yours rather than representing competition, and you should highlight this.

Length of the manuscript

Another consideration for the commissioning editor is whether the proposed length (number of words or pages, or 'extent' in publishing jargon) is appropriate. Obviously, if your book is not going to be full of solid text, but will be more of a workbook with charts and templates, etc., it will be more appropriate to describe it in terms of number of pages than number of words. Publishers may ask for a very specific extent because, for example, your book will be part of a series and all the books in the series range between 35–40,000 words. In other situations, the publisher may be quite vague, suggesting a minimum of 40,000 and a maximum of 60,000 words, for example.

It is worth bearing in mind that the number of words is not the only determinant of the number of pages. Some books may be highly illustrated, so the final length will be calculated differently. Equally, the publisher's designers and typesetters can use smaller font sizes, squeeze more lines on to the page and even put text into two columns rather than one if they want to restrict the number of pages. Alternatively, if the manuscript is somewhat short, they may use a large font and plenty of white space in their page layout.

Some publishers aim for most of their books to fall within a particular word or page extent, and if they have made this an explicit policy, they may reject your proposal on the strength of this alone if it does not fit this criterion. It is more likely, however, that if they like the idea of your book, they will ask you to expand or reduce it.

Cost is one of the reasons why publishers are so concerned about defining length at the beginning of the process and ensuring that you keep to it. The longer the manuscript, the more the book will cost to produce and the more the publisher will need to charge for it. If they feel that the length you propose is going to make the book too expensive for the target readership, they will probably suggest that you reduce it.

If you are not sure about the length to aim for, talk to the commissioning editor.

Illustrations

Illustrations can, of course, enhance a book, particularly in breaking up otherwise turgid text. Illustrative material can take many forms, from simple tables and charts to complex graphics and photographs. Most publishers will use artists to take the material you provide for diagrams, charts, etc. and produce it in the appropriate size and format for the printer, so you will not be expected to provide camera-ready artwork.

Photographs need to be of very high quality to be reproduced in a book, and can represent a significant extra cost to production, as they need to be printed on higher-quality paper than standard text in order to do them justice. You should therefore ensure that you can justify including them.

Books containing colour illustrations and photographs are significantly more expensive to produce than those printed in one colour. The number of books with colour illustrations that publishers produce varies from none to their entire list. If

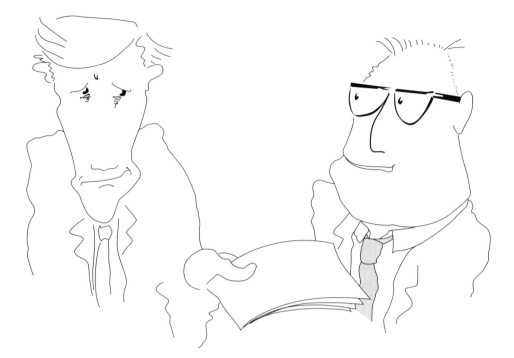

I'm sorry but it's too short

Can't you just use a larger font size?

you are approaching a publisher who rarely prints in colour, you will need some convincing arguments for including colour illustrations.

Many publishers of large books, particularly those with colour illustrations, are now producing their books in the Far East, as it is much cheaper to do so.

Sell yourself and your collaborators!

The need for a section in your proposal about you and any other authors is discussed in detail in Chapter 4. The minimum needed from a publisher's point of view is to be convinced that you and any other authors are the ideal people to write the book. They are unlikely to want to wade through a full CV, but you need to persuade them that you have the knowledge, experience and skills required for this project. Do you know enough to be credible? This is one of the questions that will be asked during the reviewing process. It does not necessarily matter that you do not have many academic qualifications or a long list of prestigious appointments. You simply need to demonstrate that what you do have is relevant to the book.

If you have published before, this is an advantage. You will probably not need to go into details about exactly what you have published. The importance of your publishing experience to the publisher is that it demonstrates you can produce coherent writing, are likely to find the time and discipline to write, can meet deadlines, can write within pre-arranged word limits, know how to correct proofs and understand something of the publishing process and an author's responsibilities.

Timescale

How you decide how long it will take to write your book and how you manage your writing time are discussed in detail in Chapters 1 and 7. How crucial it is that your book should be published at a particular time – for example, to be launched at a conference, or for a new intake of students – is something you will need to discuss with the publisher. Bear in mind that it will probably take at least five to six months from acceptance of your manuscript to publication.

Approaching your chosen publisher

Some publishers specify on their website or in printed literature how they wish to receive proposals. If not, contact your chosen publisher by phone or email in the first instance to find out whether they would be interested in receiving your proposal. Email has the advantage that you can summarise your ideas exactly as you wish without interruption. It also gives the commissioning editor more time to consider your ideas and decide how to respond. If you phone, and they are busy or in a bad mood, they may dismiss your ideas without giving them due consideration. Most publishers' websites will tell you whom to contact. If no name is given, address your email to 'the commissioning editor' and it should be forwarded to the most appropriate person.

Most professional/non-trade publishers prefer to receive a proposal for a book in the first instance, rather than a manuscript. The reason for this is that they can then work with the author to ensure that their book meets the needs of its audience. If a publisher receives a manuscript, this is less likely to be easily done.

Once you have submitted your proposal, if you don't receive any kind of response or acknowledgement after a couple of weeks, it is probably worth following it up to check that they have received it. If they have and you still do not hear anything, this is discourteous and you might question whether you would really want these people to publish your work. You might decide to write and tell them that, as you have not heard from them, you are assuming that they are not interested and are approaching another publisher. This sometimes provokes a response, and if it does not, you have not lost anything.

What you hope at this stage is that at least you will receive a friendly, positive response saying that they are interested in your proposal and are going to have it reviewed. This process is likely to take a few weeks, or sometimes even months.

The reviewing process

In-house review

Most publishers will initially review your proposal in-house, but sometimes this is done at the same time as the external review (*see* below). The internal review normally involves editorial and marketing personnel. The editorial team will consider whether and how it would fit with the current publishing programme and the other books on their list, and the marketing team will assess its sales potential. They may be asked to present their conclusions to a higher level of decision making within the organisation – even to the board of directors. This is likely to be the case if the project is large and requires substantial investment or represents a significant departure from the current publishing programme in a way that may affect future plans and budgets.

Sometimes the commissioning editor alone will be able to make an assessment and reach a positive decision without consultation. This is often the case when they are very experienced, the proposal fits well with the existing publishing programme and the author is experienced and well known to the company.

However, even when this happens, they will sometimes send the proposal for external review. This is not as part of the decision-making process on whether or not to publish, but because the reviewers' perspectives are useful adjuncts to consider.

External review

Often the publisher will wish to have your proposal reviewed by one or more independent experts in the field. Reviewers are selected on the basis of their understanding of the subject area, the market and what they might know about what else is in the pipeline from other publishers. An external reviewer who is an expert in the area may have suggestions that could enhance the book. They may have been chosen because they are likely to know whether any other authors are writing a similar book – they may even be writing it themselves! They may be well placed to assess a secondary market that the publisher is less familiar with, but that the proposed author has suggested could be interested in the book. Or perhaps they are involved in education and suggest revisions to the proposed writing style or content so that the book is more likely to be adopted as a course text.

The kinds of questions that they may be asked include the following:

- What do you consider are the scope and size of the market for this book?
- Does it have international potential?
- Who do you think might buy it?
- Does the contents list cover all the topics you would expect to see?
- What additional contents might be appropriate?
- How could the proposal be enhanced?
- How appropriate are the length, style and format as proposed for the intended audience?
- How could the book's presentation be enhanced?
- How well recognised is the author in this field? If they are not well recognised, how important do you consider this to be?
- Are you aware of any existing or forthcoming titles that might compete in this area?
- What might be the advantages of this proposed book?
- How might this proposal be improved to ensure that it has a clear advantage over competing texts?
- Would you recommend that we publish this book?

If a publisher specialises in particular fields, they may have a team of reviewers retained for the purpose of considering their proposals. If their list is somewhat more eclectic, they may consult reviewers on an ad hoc basis.

The process is usually carried out anonymously – that is, you as the aspiring author are not told the identity of the reviewer. However, you may be given some information about them, such as their job title, if it adds credibility to their views.

Publishers may ask you to recommend someone who could comment on your proposal, particularly if it has unusual aspects. Equally you may ask them to seek the views of someone whose opinion you would value but who you feel might not provide such frank feedback if you were to approach them yourself.

The reviewing process and the decision as to whether to commission your book can take from days to months. In-house meetings to consider new proposals may take place infrequently, and boards of directors may only convene monthly. Expert reviewers invariably have other things to do with their time and remuneration is negligible, often taking the form of a selection of books from the publisher's list or a book token. When this is all that is offered, the commissioning editor may be reluctant to chase the reviewer. However, they should give you some idea at the beginning of the process how long it might take, and most will not resent you contacting them from time to time to get an update on progress.

Once the feedback has been received from the reviewer, their comments will be taken into consideration with the results of the in-house review. If the conclusion is that the publisher would like to commission your book, the comments will usually be fed back to you. You may be asked to revise the proposal. You do not have to accept every suggestion, and you may wish to negotiate some points, but it is important to be flexible. The commissioning editor and their colleagues are experts in publishing and their objective views can be valuable. You have a long working relationship ahead, so it is important to get off to a good start. It will not usually be necessary to resubmit your proposal, but keep a note of agreed amendments.

You are now ready to talk about contracts and next steps.

Rejection!

There is great variation in the way that publishers respond to aspiring authors, particularly if they are rejecting them. Some can be quite brutal and/or rude, sending a curt standard letter of rejection without reason or explanation. They would probably argue that they receive so many proposals that they do not have time to respond personally to those which they do not want to pursue. Others will offer reasons for rejection, and give feedback – perhaps even suggestions for changes to the proposal and which other publishers to approach.

Rejection need not be the end. Many successful authors have been rejected at some stage. It does not mean that you cannot write a book suitable for publication. The reasons for rejection may be nothing to do with the merits of your proposal or your ability to write the book.

Should you appeal?

This depends on the reasons given for rejection. If it is the publisher's view that 'we do not feel that your proposed book fits our list', then there is no point. This is the publisher's decision based on their criteria.

However, if your proposal has been rejected on the basis of the reviewer's view that 'I do not feel there's likely to be great interest in it', and you have evidence to dispute this, then you can try an appeal. Equally, if in the reviewer's opinion the ground is already covered, but you believe that the existing books are out of date or provide a different focus, you can try! Back up your appeal with evidence. It is probably a good idea to let the commissioning editor know that you plan to appeal, in case they have decided they do not wish to commission your book whatever evidence you might provide. You can then put your efforts into reworking your proposal for another publisher.

Whatever you do, do not waste time in blaming the situation on the reviewing system, or the vagaries of commissioning editors, as this will not help. Reassess your proposal, think about why you did not manage to persuade this publisher, and get on with persuading another.

The contract or memorandum of agreement

So your proposal has been accepted and the publisher is going to publish your book. You now need to sign a contract. Most publishers' contracts are fairly standard, although some contain a lot more legal jargon than others. Some authors like to involve their solicitor in looking at their contract. This is not advisable unless the solicitor has some experience of publishing contracts, or unless you are happy to hand over lots of money to a solicitor in return for protracted discussions with your publisher, which will probably leave you in the same position as you were when you started, or without a publisher.

The contract should include the following:

- which rights over your work you grant to the publisher (i.e. format and territory)
- the date, terms and conditions for delivery of the manuscript
- the conditions for acceptance of the manuscript
- the publisher's responsibility to publish the book
- the procedure for corrections
- responsibility for obtaining and paying for copyright permissions
- royalties, other payments and statements about sales
- author's copies
- future revisions
- remainders and disposal of surplus stock
- termination of the contract.

As an example, you can find the Radcliffe Publishing Memorandum of Agreement at www.radcliffe-oxford.com.

What happens next?

How to write your book is covered in detail in Chapter 7. During this time you should keep in touch with your editor (if you have one), particularly if:

- you want to change the brief
- you want to change a co-author/contributor
- you want to add or omit a chapter
- you want to extend the deadline.

You may also want to ask for advice and feedback as you progress, particularly in the early stages of writing.

The editorial and production processes

Assuming all goes well, you submit your manuscript on time and it is accepted. Box 9.1 provides a summary of the stages from acceptance to publication, with approximate timings that apply at Radcliffe Publishing, although these will vary between publishers. They may be longer if some of the processes are carried out in the Far East.

Box 9.1 Publication schedule

1 Receipt of manuscript. Manuscript passed to commissioning editor for perusal and comment. Undetermined time period, depending on any necessary changes to be made by author. Average time period: 2 weeks–3 weeks.
2 Manuscript passed to editorial project management team. An in-house meeting is arranged to discuss issues such as title, book format, price, cover design, etc. Average time period: 2 weeks.
3 Manuscript is sent out for editing and returned along with a list of author queries. Average time period: 3 weeks.

4   Author queries sent on to author for responses. Average time period: 2 weeks–3 weeks.
5   Amendments to manuscript made in-house when query responses have been received. Manuscript sent to typesetters for preparation of page proofs. Average time period: 4 weeks.
6   Page proofs sent out to author, proofreader, indexer and foreword writer (if applicable). Further author queries raised by the proofreader are addressed at this stage. Average time period: 3 weeks.
7   Author's and proofreader's corrections amalgamated on to one set of proofs. Index checked and inserted. Average time period: 1 week.
8   Marked page proofs returned to the typesetter for preparation of revised page proofs. These are checked in-house and any further corrections are sent back to the typesetter. Average time period: 3 weeks.
9   Once final revisions have been checked, book goes to press. Cover is being printed at this stage. Average time period: 4 weeks.

The average time from receipt of manuscript to publication is 6 months.

The first step in the production process once your manuscript has been accepted is that the publisher will decide on the title, format, layout, text design, cover design, price and schedule. Your input into these discussions and negotiations is discussed in Chapter 11.

Copy editing

Your manuscript will then be passed to a copy editor. Usually the publisher will have asked for an electronic and hard (i.e. paper-based) copy. Some copy editors edit on screen, but others still use hard copy. Their job is to read the text in great detail, check grammar and spelling, ensure that everything that needs to be is referenced, and that all references provided are complete. They will also assess the content for consistency, which is particularly important if you have a number of contributors writing from different perspectives and with different writing styles. They will check that acronyms are spelt out in full at first mention and that jargon and complicated terms are explained.

Their other task is to mark up the manuscript for the typesetter, indicating the hierarchy of headings, which material should be put into bulleted lists, where tables and figures should be placed, etc. Meanwhile, an artist will be redrawing diagrams and other illustrations to fit the format of the book.

When the copy editor has finished going through the manuscript, they will compile a list of queries for the author. These may be sent to the author for their response and further revisions of the manuscript by the copy editor before the manuscript goes to the typesetter, or they may be kept for the proofreading stage.

Typesetting, proofreading and indexing

The manuscript is then sent to the typesetter, who will follow the template provided by the publisher for the page layout and font style and size.

The next thing that you will see is page proofs – your manuscript presented on A4 sheets showing how it will look in the final book version.

The publisher should alert you to when you will be receiving the proofs, and will ask you to check them for errors and return the corrected proofs by a certain date. The timescale for this is usually negotiable. If you are the editor you may check the whole manuscript yourself, or you may organise the individual contributors to check their own chapters and then collate all their responses yourself.

At this stage, the publisher wants you to check the proofs to ensure that they are correct. This is not an opportunity to rewrite your text. Obviously, if something has happened that means that the text needs updating, you should update it, but only essential changes should be made. At this stage, every change – even the addition of a comma or deletion of an apostrophe – will incur a charge from the typesetter of at least 75 pence. But of course the publisher wants the final version to be as up to date as possible.

At the same time that you are reading and correcting the proofs, the publisher will usually employ a proofreader to check them for typographical errors. They will also have sent the proofs to a professional indexer for them to compile an index for the book, although there are some publishers who expect the author to provide the index. This is another reason why substantial changes are difficult and expensive to incorporate at this stage. If they affect the pagination, the index will need to be changed.

When your corrections and those of the proofreader have been received, the publisher collates them and returns the proofs to the typesetter. Unless the corrections are substantial, you will not usually see the proofs again; they will be checked by the publisher.

Meanwhile, the publisher will have approved the cover design, and the back-cover copy will have been prepared. Sometimes these will be discussed with you.

The book then goes to press and several weeks later is published.

Chapter 10

The publisher's side: finance, marketing and promotion

Gregory Moxon

This chapter gives you some idea of what a publisher can do to promote your book, and how you can help them in that process. It includes a brief explanation of the costs underlying a book's publication, and how the money from a typical sale is split. This should give you a better idea of the level of resources it is reasonable to expect a publisher to devote to promoting your book, so that you can agree with them what is the best mix of activities for your particular title.

After discussing the kind of information that publishers want from their authors, and how book details such as title and price are set, the chapter outlines the various activities that publishers typically carry out in promoting a book, and how you as the author can have an influence in making these activities successful.

The financial pie

Figure 10.1 provides an overview of the various costs incurred in publication. When a book is bought, the price paid is typically sliced up to cover the following:

- bookshop discount
- sales representation cost
- packing and delivery
- order processing and accounting
- marketing
- warehousing
- printing
- typesetting
- editorial
- author royalties.

Overall, there is a mixture of direct costs and overheads (staff salaries, office running costs), all of which have to be paid entirely out of the revenues from the sales of the books.

The costs of editing the text might be absorbed within the publisher's overheads as part of their salaried staff, or might be paid directly to freelance editors. The same applies to the other editorial costs of proofreading and indexing.

There may be various costs involved in using copyright images such as photographs, either within the book or on its cover, and diagrams and illustrations may need to be redrawn. Any contributors' fees have to be paid, where agreed. If for some reason your book quotes another work extensively, it may be that you will have to license that material from its publisher, and payment will have to be made, either as a fee or as extra royalties from sales revenues. Sometimes a book can benefit from having additional information (such as forms, templates, data or audiovisual material) included on a CD-ROM or DVD mounted in the book. All of these factors can affect the price that the publisher calculates they must charge for the book, which in turn affects how attractive the book is to its market, and its viability. Consider these matters thoroughly when preparing your book proposal.

The typesetting costs, the physical costs of materials such as paper and ink, and the printing process, also have to be borne. There are numerous other less tangible charges that publishers face. When a book is printed, it has to be stored. Whether this is at a publisher's own warehouse or at a distributor's, this costs money. Each time a book is sent out, it costs money for the labour to pack and despatch it, for the materials used to wrap it and for the delivery itself. There are the back-office costs of the ordering system – invoicing and stock control – without which records could not be properly kept or royalties accurately paid.

Publishers may employ their own team of sales representatives to sell books to bookshops, or they may contract this function out to independent sales people or sales teams. The publisher either incurs an overhead cost for salaries and related expenditure such as travel, or pays a commission that is partly or wholly based on sales revenues. The bookshops themselves retain a portion of the price of each book they sell, in the form of their trade discount. This varies according to commercial arrangements and the type of publishing, but is usually at least a quarter and can be over half of the retail price of the book.

As the resources available to your publisher to promote your work arise from just one slice of this 'pie' (*see* Figure 10.1), you and they need to work closely together to ensure that the most is made from it!

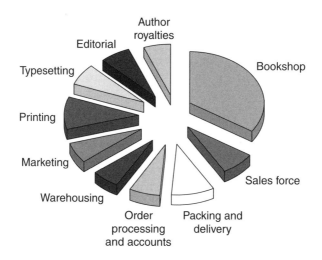

Figure 10.1 Where the money goes from the sale of a book.

What you can tell your publisher

When you sign your contract or when you submit your manuscript, your publisher may send you some form of questionnaire, to help you to provide them with other details they will find useful in marketing and promoting your book. Tell the marketing team at your publisher about the following:

- how you want to be described (your affiliations)
- why the book is needed
- the target readers
- competing books
- useful contacts (organisations, journals, conferences, etc.).

The details might include your job title or professional affiliations, in the form in which you wish them to be used when describing you in reviews and in advertising material. These details should be brief rather than comprehensive, as space is limited.

In due course the publisher will produce a blurb – that is, a promotional description of the book. This will be used on the book cover and may be further adapted in leaflets, catalogues or advertisements promoting the book. The author's questionnaire will often include a space for you to describe the book briefly, and this is a useful opportunity for you to influence the blurb and ensure that it contains what you see as the key points. Brevity is valuable. It is not necessary to mention all the topics that the book covers, or the conclusions that it reaches. The most useful information you can provide is to establish why the book is needed – that is, to identify what has previously been missing among the available resources in this field. Specify the readership as you see it. If you are able to define your target readers tightly and in order of importance, this will be much appreciated.

The author's questionnaire will probably give you a chance to mention any competing books. Provide the publisher with as much information as you can. Although they will probably already be aware of other works in the field, they are not experts in your area of study, and may not fully appreciate why your work complements or extends other material. The publisher needs to be able to communicate why your book has appeal. In particular, they need to make these points clearly to bookshops, and you can help them to do this properly.

You may have covered a lot of this ground previously in your book proposal, but there are good reasons for going over it again now. You are now providing the information to a different group of people within the publishing organisation – to the sales and marketing staff rather than their editorial colleagues – and things may have changed since you first proposed your book. You may have changed jobs, new books in the field may have appeared, and your book may have altered significantly during the writing process. This is your chance to ensure that these changes are noted.

You may have an opportunity here to tell the publisher about any key contacts, organisations, journals or events that you feel may be useful in promoting your book. Do make sure that you mention them. Your publisher may already be aware of some, but never assume this!

Setting the details

To avoid later difficulties and disappointments, around the time your book enters your publisher's editorial and production process, check that you are happy with their decisions on the following:

- the title
- the form of your name as it will appear in the book
- the price of the book
- the appearance of the book, such as the cover design.

When your manuscript has been submitted and accepted and enters the publisher's editorial and production system, many publishers will have a meeting at which it will be discussed and various details finalised. The publisher may involve you in some of these. There will be final agreement on the book's title and, if it has one, its subtitle. The number by which it is identified by libraries and bookshops around the world, which is known as its ISBN (International Standard Book Number), is confirmed, along with any restrictions to the work's sale in any formats or territories. These might arise because of other authorial arrangements you may have, or because of certain copyright material you have reproduced in your book. Your name is confirmed in the form that it will appear in the book and on promotional material (e.g. with your first name and any middle initials as you wish them to appear). Foreword writers may be decided on or suggested. The recommended price of the book is set, and a brief for the cover design may be agreed.

You may have views on some of these points. If you have not had an opportunity to air them in your author's questionnaire, make sure that you tell your publisher about your views when you submit your manuscript. Your publisher will want to accommodate your opinions as much as possible, although this may not always be feasible. For example, your view of the ideal price for the book may be the one that makes it most affordable, whereas in some circumstances your publisher may feel that a higher price makes better commercial sense, even if it excludes some groups of readers. You may have a particular idea in mind for the cover, which may encapsulate key ideas of the book in some way. Your publisher may agree, or they may feel that it detracts from what they see as the main purpose of the cover, which is to attract potential readers and arouse interest. You may have a particular image that you would like to be used, but if the publisher has to pay for it, this may prove to be more expensive than they feel is justified.

Most of the time, you and the publisher should agree without too much difficulty – after all, you both want to make a successful book! The main thing is to finalise these details, which are then circulated externally, and are thereafter difficult to amend.

Sales channels

The various major channels through which publishers aim to gain sales include the following:

- the book trade
- direct sales to readers
- conferences and meetings

- special sales
- electronic/online sales.

Good publishers ensure that they use various channels, although different publishers concentrate on some more than others.

Publishers often specialise, concentrating on particular subjects or genres, or focusing on certain types of reader (e.g. professional, academic or general public). Consequently, some may be better at selling into academic bookshops than into consumer (high-street) bookshops. Some publishers may have excellent shop presence but do little direct marketing. Some large publishers might be strong in all of these channels, but if they have a correspondingly large publishing programme, your book might not receive the individual sales and marketing attention that you would like, and it may be lost among too many other titles.

Ideally you are working with a publisher who:

- is used to targeting the kind of reader at whom your book is primarily aimed
- has efficient systems in place for reaching them
- has a reasonable number of similar but not directly competing books with which yours can be grouped in order to maximise the range and cost-effectiveness of the sales and marketing activities.

Talk with potential publishers frankly about what they see as their strengths and weaknesses in these areas.

Your author contract will specify the percentage of your royalties, and you may receive a different percentage from some types of sale because of the costs that the publisher incurs there.

Bookshops

First, there is the book trade. Factors that affect how successfully your book will be sold into the book trade include the following:

- the reach of the publisher's representation (whether their sales staff visit the full range of bookshops that are likely to be interested in stocking your book, and how good their relationships are with key shops and trade buyers)
- the volume of books that they present
- how they see your book within that overall list.

Ideally, you want your book to be a significant highlight in a credible list of titles to which a bookshop must pay attention.

Bookshop buyers only allow publishers' representatives very limited time to spend on each title they present. Therefore sales reps need a few key points to relay to the bookshop buyer, to enable them to make an appropriate purchasing decision. It is not always necessary for them to explain what your book is about – it may be more important for the bookshop buyer to know, for example, that there is proven demand for the subject which your book addresses. Booksellers do not necessarily share your love of your subject – nor do they need to – they just need to be convinced that their customers will.

The role of publishers and their representatives is to influence bookshops, which of course make their own commercial decisions on what to stock and when. Generally, a bookshop will only stock copies of a particular book on a single subject shelf. This can be frustrating for publishers and authors, but makes sense for the shops. So if your book has relevance in more than one subject area, be clear about which one is the most important, and make sure that your publisher knows this and will tell the shops. If a customer cannot find a book on the shelf where they expected it to be, the bookshop staff can find where it is stocked in their shop. However, it is important that the book is placed where the customers most likely to be interested in it will browse.

The book trade includes not only bookshops, but also wholesalers (who are intermediaries, selling to smaller shops), library supply companies and online suppliers. If your book has potential for sales internationally, you will also want to consider how well your publisher reaches those markets. This might be through their own international offices or through a network of distributors and agents, and via foreign publishers to whom they sell publishing rights, including exhibiting at major international book fairs such as that held annually at Frankfurt.

Direct sales

A second sales channel involves selling direct to the customer. The importance of this varies enormously depending on the type of book and the particular publisher's usual practice. Often, for a book written by a professional to inform and help fellow professionals, sales direct to readers can form a very significant proportion of the total. How well publishers handle these sales varies enormously, too. As an author, you will be interested in how active the publisher is in direct marketing, and how responsive and efficient they are in dealing with enquiries and orders from individual customers, compared with the way they work with the book trade.

You may find that, as a professional, you have opportunities to reach your colleagues and inform them about your book yourself. For example, you may have speaking engagements, give presentations, attend conferences, and so on. You may be able to arrange for advertising leaflets about your book to be distributed to conference delegates. And you may be able to inform your publisher about many other promotional opportunities, even if you will not be there in person. If your publisher is responsive to your requests for such leaflets, your book will benefit considerably. However, do be aware that your publisher must consider the cost of producing these leaflets and other marketing material, which has to be proportionate to the likely resulting sales.

You may have access to relevant mailing lists or email bulletins sent out by groups within your network. Work with your publisher to make the most of these.

You may wish to sell copies of your book yourself at such events, or at other nodes in your professional network. Your author contract may well specify the discount at which you are entitled to purchase copies.

Meetings, conferences and courses

Conferences and professional meetings are excellent places for your publisher to display your book and sell copies wherever possible. Sometimes publishers attend these events themselves and sometimes they work with third parties, such as specialist travelling bookshops. You will want to consider how important these are for your particular books, and how effective your publisher is at achieving exposure here. Many publishers are diligent in gathering information on relevant events and pursuing opportunities to market or sell their books there, but do not assume that a publisher will have heard about a particular meeting or conference. If you know about one, tell your publisher in plenty of time for them to make suitable arrangements. Several months in advance is not too soon!

As well as finding ways to sell books to individual customers, publishers may also be able to sell multiple copies to organisations. In healthcare, for example, there are numerous bodies that might find a particular book relevant and important to their activities. They may wish to disseminate it widely among their staff or stakeholders. Publishers will generally be pleased to arrange special discounts for multiple-copy orders to facilitate this. If you belong to such an organisation, and can bring such an order to the publisher along with your proposal, it is likely to be even more warmly received!

You may be aware of, or you may even run, a course for which your book could be essential reading. Perhaps your book could be supplied to each course participant, with the cost of the book built into the price of the course. A regular guaranteed stream of such sales helps a book to become a lasting success.

Special sales

A further route for books is what many publishers call **special sales**. These are sales to organisations, often commercial companies, which will use the books as part of their own activities. For example, they may use them promotionally as special offers, or as free promotional items. In healthcare, pharmaceutical companies use books in this way as gifts to doctors and their colleagues or as educational support material. They may buy hundreds or thousands of copies, often at a significant discount, and they may want a special cover on the book to make it more suitable for the use they have in mind.

This can be the most effective channel of all in getting the book into the hands of readers, simply because of the large quantities involved. In general this does not involve any compromise in terms of content or authorial independence, and your contract should ensure that changes to your work could not be made without your approval. You should be reassured that any such sales would not damage the way you or your work are perceived, but if you have any reservations you should ensure that any restrictions are clearly laid out in your author's contract. This would affect how your publisher assesses the commercial potential of your book, and could alter their decision to publish it. On the other hand, you may have contacts with potential special sales customers such as drug company representatives. If you do, tell your publisher and pass those potential customers' details on.

Electronic media

Professional books are increasingly becoming available to read in electronic form online, and publishers are working with partners in this evolving area to ensure that developments take place in ways that benefit readers, publishers and authors. Your author contract should allow for this use, and should specify the royalty percentage you will receive.

Marketing and promotion

The marketing process has already begun, by ensuring that the book is best suited to its market with its price being set, its title finalised and its cover design decided. Information about the book is disseminated to the book trade, and various trade promotions may be agreed that include your book.

Work closely with your publisher to help them to market your book in the following ways:

- book-trade marketing
- marketing direct to potential readers
- events
- publicity and PR
- networking.

Launch events can be useful both in generating sales and in seeding awareness of the book among influential colleagues. These can be hosted by a relevant organisation, or they can be held at a place of work or an academic centre. Sometimes they can form part of the programme of a relevant conference or other meeting. For professional books where colleagues in a particular region may have special interest in the appearance of a book, an event at a suitable bookshop may be preferable to attract a wider audience. Your publisher can work with appropriate bookshop partners to arrange this, if you wish.

Look back earlier in this chapter to recall how disseminating information to attract direct sales, and ensuring that your book is visible at appropriate meetings and conferences, can be vital to its success. Take every opportunity to talk with your publisher about these opportunities.

Your publisher will in all probability go to considerable lengths to obtain free publicity for your book through press and media exposure. Depending on your subject, this may be entirely focused on professional journals, or it may also include some element of general media, such as national newspapers. However, for the latter to be realistically achievable, there has to be a clear story of interest to the newspaper's ordinary readers as well as to fellow professionals. Sometimes this may not be the same theme that is of most importance for professional colleagues. This is not in itself a problem, as whatever attracts interest in the book is worthwhile. Perhaps you can help by generating interesting stories.

There is a wide range of potential activities in professional journals that can create publicity for your book. Book reviews are a valuable source of information to potential readers, and you should agree with your publisher the list of journals to which your book should be offered for review. You may already have personal contacts with certain editors or journalists, in which case you should discuss these with your publisher, as an approach might be more successful coming from you rather than from them.

In addition, some publications may wish to publish extracts from your work, either as stand-alone articles or in a series. You can work with your publisher to select the most appropriate sections and to decide on the proportion of the book that can be used in this way. It is often sensible to view this as a promotional activity rather than as a potential source of revenue, and your publisher may also agree with the journal to give away copies of your book as prizes in a competition, or to tie in a special offer for your book to readers of the journal.

Some publications may wish to interview you on themes related to your book, and as an active professional in your field you may have opportunities to write articles on similar topics from time to time. When this happens, remember to tell your publisher well ahead of time, so that they can arrange for publicity for your book to run alongside the article. Where appropriate, it is sensible for you to include the right to such publicity in your agreement with the journal. Always ensure that you are credited as the author of a relevant book, using wording which you can agree with the publisher, to ensure that readers can easily find ways to purchase copies.

Lastly, as an active professional you will be part of professional networks and may be involved in courses or other aspects of continuing professional development where your book may be of use. This more personal aspect of promotion can be hugely important to the success of your book, so do not be shy of using opportunities here! Tell your publisher about all the activities you are involved in, and put them in touch with key contacts in cases where it would be more appropriate for your publisher, rather than you, to make arrangements.

Good publishers will continue to work on a book for as long as it has a use, not just in a quick burst around the time of publication. Similarly, once your book is published and the first flush of activity is over, you should not forget about it either and assume that there is nothing more to be done. Cultivate it like a flower – you have planted it successfully, but now it must be continually nourished if it is to blossom fully. Keep talking with your publisher, letting them know about possible opportunities for further promotion, and asking them what more you can do to help. With careful and continuing attention your book will inform and influence established and new readers for a long time to come.

Chapter 11

Improving your writing technique

Ruth Chambers

When you start out writing, you are usually blind to most of your faults. Initially, you perceive that any negative feedback which you receive means that people do not understand what you are trying to say, or that they have not bothered to read all of your report or article. As you spend hours sweating over an overheated keyboard, you realise that you have a lot to learn if you are to emulate other people who seemingly write quickly and succinctly and with ease. You face up to the choice you have to make. You could carry on in a low-key amateurish way churning out the occasional report or article that publishers desperate for copy will accept. Or you could master the technique of writing for the particular field and target readers with whom you want to communicate. So how can you do the latter?

You do not necessarily have to develop a trademark style for one type of writing or readership. You might experiment with writing poetry or fiction at the same time as you develop your skills in writing academic books for health professionals, or health-promoting articles for the general public, for instance. You might find that experimenting with a range of different writing outputs helps you to find the style you enjoy and the particular readership most suited to your preferred type of writing. This links back to your reasons for writing in the first place, as covered in Chapter 1.

If you are primarily writing to inform patients about the actions to take in order to regain or sustain their health, then you want to develop a simple type of prose that is easy to read and understand. If your main reason for writing is to accelerate your academic career, then you will write in a manner that conforms to the requirements of reputable peer-reviewed journals.

Enrol on a writing course

There are a great variety of writing courses available. You could register on a course at your local college or university, if you are interested in creative writing or journalism. You could attend a writing course for those in the NHS focused on specific areas such as academic writing or editing, at different levels of expertise, from beginners to more experienced writers (*see*, for example, www.timalbert. co.uk). The most popular courses run by Tim Albert Training include effective writing, writing a journal article, editing medical journals and medical journalism.

Much of what you learn on such a course comes from your interaction with the other participants. You learn from sharing your material, reviewing each others' work, hearing other participants' reflections and receiving their insights, as Jackie did when she participated in the writing course described in Box 11.1. You also observe how the tutors or facilitators perform as writers. At the completion of the course, you can evaluate the relevance of their tips to you and your individual circumstances or preferences.

Box 11.1 Tale end of a course

Jackie went on a week-long residential creative writing course in rural Wales when she was starting out as a writer and had yet to determine which style and focus suited her. The other 12 'students' came from all walks of life. Some had just started trying to write for publication, while others wanted to improve or diversify. Two renowned writers of fiction facilitated the course and acted as role models for the group. Some of their tips were relevant to Jackie – such as carrying a notebook in which to jot down observations and reflections that might be incorporated in future writing. Some of their advice was less feasible – like shutting yourself up in a room for six weeks with a continual supply of whisky until the book manuscript was drafted (Jackie did not like the taste of whisky, and there was the little matter of her day job as a GP to think about, too). Every evening the course participants read out the extracts of their work of which they were most proud, or writing by others that they admired. By the end of the week Jackie felt that such creative writing was not her forte, while others present had honed their talent.

Read all about it

Tim Albert's website carries a lot of information about recommended books that you might find helpful (e.g. a book on how to write tables clearly). It is constantly evolving, so is worth checking at intervals to see what is new. There are sections on the writing process, on medical writing and publishing in journals, and on grammar and style. As a writer it is worth investing time in reading other people's tips and guidance to give you insight into the kinds of mistakes that other people make and that you would, of course, always avoid.

Join a writers' association, group or society

Support and self-help groups, or organisations for aspiring writers, can be local or national. Some are specifically for those working in, or retired from, the health setting. The Society of Authors has a medical writers' group (www. societyofauthors.net). It was formed in 1979 to offer practical help and advice to medical authors, and to provide a forum for discussion on issues that affect medical writers. It has a quarterly journal, *The Author*. The Society will advise on your contract from a publisher and on copyright issues. If you belong to the Society this gives you automatic membership of the Authors Licensing and Collecting Society (ALCS), which collects and distributes monies received for photocopying and other fees.

The Society of Medical Writers (SOMW) was established in 1985, and holds one or two residential meetings per year for health professional members with various themes (www.somw.org.uk). Their regular magazine *The Writer* provides an opportunity for members to publish their work, which ranges from poetry to reports, and from short stories to book reviews. The members' database is publicly available to publishers of news-sheets and books, and sometimes writers are approached to write an article or other material because of the special interests or expertise they have declared. The workshops give members an opportunity to chat to successful authors, join in training, and listen to publishers or literary agents or well-published writers speaking about their experiences and insights, as Ruth found in Box 11.2.

Box 11.2 Learning the craft

Ruth joined the SOMW when she had started to write the occasional article for the medical press. She found the residential meetings inspiring, and learned to craft her writing for her intended medical readership. The SOMW workshops gave her the confidence to write to editors of GP newspapers to suggest that they commission articles on topics she briefly described. She began to understand what was the key to shaping her material for the market – matched to the interests and objectives of the publication. For instance, the 'free to GPs' weekly newspapers pay for themselves by selling advertising space, mainly to pharmaceutical companies. Articles that make GPs feel good are more likely to be commissioned or accepted than pieces that show GPs in a bad light, admonish them or generally depress them.

Some organisations encourage their members to develop relevant writing skills, although their remit is far wider. For example, university academics working in education and research relevant to primary care belong to the Society for Academic Primary Care (www.sapc.ac.uk). The Society's scientific meeting always has writing workshops, although if you're looking for workshops on creative writing this is not the place to find them – unless you cynically believe that academics are trying to make more of the findings of their research studies by creative writing than the scientific base supports!

Others focus on niche areas of writing. For instance, Medics4Media provides a support and information service or network for members who publish their work or speak on television or other broadcasting outlets (www.medics4media.com). They may approach members with opportunities to engage with the media.

Participating in any special interest writers' association or local writing club will give you the chance to obtain feedback on your work. Reading and critiquing other people's writing will enable you to see what works and what does not, and you may be able to develop a more marketable style as a result. You will enjoy writing 20-word sentences with simple words rather than the convoluted lengthy prose that you churned out when you first started writing.

Book reviews: yours and others

If you have a senior job, or a post in an organisation such as a deanery, university or professional association, then you might be approached to write a book review, even if you are not an established writer. If you accept, you usually get to keep the book, and occasionally a publisher will pay you a nominal fee as well. Your main reason for reading the book and writing the review is not for a monetary reward. It should be to give a view that reflects the perspective of your background and something of why you have been chosen by the publisher as a suitable reviewer.

This is your chance to really concentrate on the scope, relevance and accuracy of the content, the nature of the enticements (or deterrents) for the reader, the readability of the material and how balanced and coherent it is. You can learn a lot from thinking about how the authors or editors approached topics in the book. Have they been successful in engaging the reader or stimulating action? And how did they achieve this result? If the book provokes negative feelings in you, puzzle out why that is, and how a different approach might have worked better. You can critique the balance between straight text and boxes or illustrations. Undertaking book reviews helps you to learn to make your own writing richer and more to the point.

Writing book reviews is an art. You have to be pithy but at the same time do justice to the book. Avoid making cheap jibes at the author's expense. You will find that they will come back to haunt and embarrass you. You might next meet them on an interview panel for that post that you really want to get, or they might review a book of yours or be able to take revenge in other ways. However, you should also avoid writing a sycophantic review without any substance. People who buy or use a poorly written book on your insincere or casual recommendation will remember the false lead you gave them and rate your critical powers just as poorly.

Read any reviews about your own published books. You could consign ones that displease you to the waste-paper basket, but it is better to take a more rounded view. The book reviewer may have exaggerated some of the weaknesses to make more of an article of the review, or they may have misinterpreted the purpose of the book, or have a completely different perspective on the subject. Sometimes you will wonder whether the reviewer actually read the book, especially when there are complaints that you have omitted material that is included. (Indeed, from having edited book reviews, Gill is convinced that some reviewers do not read the whole book.) Compare the various perspectives on your work from different reviewers, and reflect on them. Discuss the review(s) with other co-authors or writing colleagues to get the ratings in proportion, and decide what you can learn that will improve your future writing.

Experiment with various types of writing and different readership groups

The more you experiment with different types of writing, the more naturally you will craft your writing to the most appropriate type of output, whether it is a short article or a sizeable book manuscript. You could even try ghost writing, whereby someone commissions you to write articles or a book based on someone else's published work or verbal material, which purports to be written by them. It will be a challenge writing in someone else's expected style rather than your own.

You might undertake a strengths, weaknesses, opportunities and threats (SWOT) analysis of the range of your writing prowess in order to probe further into your abilities as a writer and your preferred technique. Work your way through the categories, and then discuss your responses with someone who knows you and your attempts to write well. You might end up with something like the content of the four quadrants of the SWOT analysis shown in Box 11.3 in your preliminary brainstorming.

Box 11.3 Example of an analysis of your strengths, weaknesses, opportunities and threats (SWOT) in relation to writing and your technique

Strengths	Weaknesses
• Lots of experience working in health setting – lots to write about • Versatile – can write articles on different topics • Successfully edited a book with ten chapter contributors – good book reviews	• Gave up submitting book proposals as solo author, after first two attempts were turned down two years ago • Only writes articles for one newspaper – have become fixed in same mould • Cannot bear to read own work in print, as feel that work is not really good enough
Opportunities	**Threats**
• Attended writing workshop and met established author who has proposed that you co-author book together • Workshop covered writing for publication in academic journal – will now try higher-profile journal when writing up current research project	• Colleagues have muttered unhelpful feedback about articles – 'trust (you) to make a simple thing complicated' – so you are thinking of quitting writing articles • Your mother is becoming demented and requires more support and care, reducing your personal time for writing

---

So the last stage of your SWOT analysis is to review all four quadrants, realise the opposing drivers and pressures, and formulate an action plan. In the example in Box 11.3, you might resolve to focus on doing academic writing in work time as a priority for improving and practising your writing technique in the short term, while facing up to the need to sort out and to some extent provide care for your mother.

Action stations

The most important way of improving your writing is to write and constantly look at ways that you can do it better. A book is a presentation of your ideas, like a performance or a concert, and a rehearsed and polished product is better than the first one that you did. The feedback which you receive helps you to strive towards perfection. Just **write**, keep on and on writing, and try again.

Index

Page numbers in *italic* refer to tables and figures.

abbreviations 41, 82–3
acknowledgements 78
acronyms 82–3
activity boxes 76
Adobe Illustrator 85
Advanced Medical Publishing 52
alignment 81
American Psychological Association (APA)
   citation style 84
anecdotes 77
apostrophes 72, 89
article writing 6
author queries 72, 101
author royalties 42, 104, 107
author types
  'expert' 13
  'novice' 14
  personality issues 25
  see also sole authorship
Authors Licensing and Collecting Society
   (ALCS) 114

back cover copy 102
  promotional material 105
back-office costs 104
Beaconsfield Publishers 52
Blackwell Publishers 50
BMJ Books 50
'boilerplate' terms 58
book fairs 108
book promotion 29–30, 72–3, 105, 108
  author/s input 105–6
  costs 104
  sales channels 106–9
  sales representatives 104
  time allowances 4, *33*
book proposals
  aims 37
  approaching publishers 37–41
  content guidance 38–41
  examples *42–7*
  publisher requirements 54, 92
  rejections 54, 99
  review systems 97–9

  and sample chapters 41
book reviews 115–16
book sales
  agent involvement 59
  costs 104, *104*
  direct channels 108
  meetings and conference 108–9
  online promotions 109
  pricing structures 103–4, 106
  promotional material 105–6
  shops 107–8
  special sales 109
book series 14–15, 91, 94
book titles 15–16, 92
book types 17–21
  historical accounts 21
  multi-authored 25–30
  narratives 21
  personal view points 17
  reference works 21
  research-based 18–19
  serial publications 14–15
  sole-authored 26–7, *27*, 30–3, *32*
  synopsis 20
  textbooks 19–20
  toolkits 20
bookshops 104, 107–8
boxes
  numbering systems 84
  see also activity boxes
brackets 82
brief outlines 20
  layouts 77
buddies 67
bullet points 81

CAB International 52
capital letters 80
cartoons 85
case histories 21
  permissions 85
charitable organisation publishing 50
The Chicago Manual of Style 84
co-author listings 78–9

co-authored writing
  advantages and disadvantages *32*
  contributors role 31–3, *32, 33*
  editors role 25–30, *33*
  share of royalties 42, 104
colour illustrations 94–6
commissioning editors 92
  see also publishers
contracts 99–100
  fixed 59
  negotiable 58
contributing authors 21–3
contributor listings 78–9
copy editing 72, 101
copyright notifications 78
Corel Draw 85
cover design 100, 102
creative writing courses 113–14

delayed submissions, authors 31
design and layout 75–90
  illustration and graphics 85, 94–6
  matching to book type 77
  publisher requirements 29, 41–2, 71
direct sales 108

editing co-authored books 25–30
  advantages and disadvantages *27*
  project timetables *30, 33*
  skills and qualities 25–6
editing own manuscripts 71
  time allowances 4
editorial and production processes 100–2
  mistakes and corrections 102
  proofreading 101–2
  typesetting 101
electronic media 109
The Elements of Style (Strunk and White) 90
Elsevier Science
  imprints 51
  proposal guidance 39–40
end matter 78
EndNote 29, 84
equations 84
exercise and physical activities 65, 66
'expert' authors 13
external reviews 97–9

fiction writing 58
figures and illustrations 85
  numbering 84
financial considerations, costs of
  production 103–4, *104*

first-person accounts 21
fonts 63, 80
format design 69–71, 80–1
  publisher requirements 29, 41–2, 71
forwards 78, 106
Fowler's Modern English Usage (Allen) 90
front material 78

generic names 82
'get-out' clauses 58
glossaries 16
grammar and punctuation 72, 81–3,
  89–90
  active vs. passive language 87–8
  pronoun use 88
graphics 85, 94–6, 101

Harvard referencing system 84
headings 80, 101
historical accounts 21
  layouts 77
house styles 29, 41–2, 71
humour 16, 85
hyphenation 81

ideas 69
  and writers block 66–7
illustrations 85, 94–6, 101
  numbering 84
in-house reviews 97
indexes 78, 102
ISBNs (International Standard Book
  Numbers) 55, 106

jargon 41, 86–7, 88–9

language and terminology 15–17, 41,
  86–7, 88–9
Latin names 82
lay readership 15–16
layout *see* design and layout
legends 84
length of manuscript 42, 94
line drawings 85, 94
Lippincott Williams & Wilkins 52
lists 81
literary agents 38
  benefits and drawbacks 59
  finding 61
  key roles 57–9

McGraw Hill 54
Manson Publishing 54

manuscript length 42, 94
manuscript presentation 71, 100–2
market research 37, 92–4
  identifying competitors 93–4
marketing books 9, 37, 92–6, 110–11
  literary agents role 58–9
  see also book promotion; book sales
mathematical equations 84
Medics4Media 115
memorandums of agreement 99–100
  see also contracts
mind maps 69, *70*
mistakes and corrections 102
Modern Language Association (MLA)
    citation style 84–5
motivation to write 1–3
  personal fulfilment 9
  professional advancement 6, 8–9
  professional role expectations 9–10
  sharing information 5, 8–9
multi-author books
  advantages and disadvantages *32*
  contributors role 21–3, 31–3, *32*
  editors role 25–30
  share of royalties 42, 104
Myers–Briggs personality profile 25

narrative accounts 21
  layouts 77
  permissions 85
novice writers 14

online sales 109
opening paragraphs 79–80
outlines and synopses 20
  see also book proposals
overseas publication 51
Oxford University Press 54
  proposal guidance 40

page proofs 101
paragraphs
  opening 79
  organisation 79–80
permissions 85
personal accounts 21
personality factors
  and authorship 25
  and editing 25–6
Pharmaceutical Press 50
pharmaceuticals 82
photographs 85, 94–6
plagiarism 18

Plain English website 88
planning sessions 67, *68*
'polishing' text 71
prefaces 78
prepositions 90
pricing structures 103–4, 106
projects as books 20
promotional 'blurb' 105
pronouns 88
proofreading 72
  making corrections 102
  publication schedules *101*, 102
  time allowances *4*
proposals *see* book proposals
publication schedules *100–1*
publishers
  attitudes towards proposals 92
  commissioning considerations 91–2
  identifying market gaps 91–2
  review activities 97
  see also publishing houses
publisher's guidelines 54
publisher's lists 52
publishing houses
  author approaches to 37–41, 96–7
  choice considerations 49–54
  financial and cost aspects 103–4, *104*
  house style 29, 71
  professional affiliations 49–50
  review processes 97–9
  size considerations 52–3
  subsidiaries and imprints 51–2

queries 72, 101
quotation marks 82
quotes 81

Radcliffe Publishing 29, 52
  contractual agreements 100
RAEs (research assessment exercises) 9
readership
  general interest 15–16
  specialist/professional 16–17
reference books 21
  layouts 77
Reference Manager 29, 84
references 84–5
  checking 101
RefViz 29
rejections 54, 99
  appeals 99
'requirements for authors' 54
research, time allowances 4

research thesis 18–19
reviews 115–16
Routledge 52
    proposal guidance 40
Royal College of General Practitioners
    50
royalties 42, 104, 107
RSM Press 50

sales figures 59
    see also book promotion; book sales
self-publishing 54–6
    paying for help 56
    practicalities and printing 55–6
sentences
    active vs. passive 87–8
    length 85–6
series production 14–15, 91, 94
Society for Academic Primary Care (SAPC)
    115
Society of Authors 62, 114
Society of Medical Writers (SOMW)
    114–15
software packages
    illustrations and graphics 85
    word-processing 63–4, 71
sole authorship 26–7, *27*, 30–3, *32*
    time allowances 3–5, 30–1
special sales 109
specialist readership 16–17
spelling 82–3
split infinitives 90
style *see* design and layout; writing styles
support organisations 62, 114–15
symbols 83
synopsis 20
    layouts 77

tables 77, 83–4
Taylor & Francis, imprints 52
text formatting 63–4, 71, 80–1
textbooks 19–20
    layouts 77
TFM publishing 54
thesis and dissertations 18–19
Tim Albert Training 113–14
timescales
    agreeing terms 41
    for editing books 27–30, *30*

for manuscript preparation *4*, 30–1, *33*,
    33–5, 41
for publishing *100–1*
title page 78
titles
    of books 15–16, 92
    of tables/figures 84
toolkits 20
topical subjects 17
trade names 82
typefaces *see* fonts
typesetting 101
    correction charges 102
    costs 104, *104*

USA citation styles 84–5
USA spelling 82

Vancouver referencing style 29, 84
'vanity publishing' 56
voice recognition software 64

wholesalers 108
word counts 42, 94
word-processing packages
    format and fonts 63–4
    publisher requirements 71
work schedules *see* publication schedules;
        writing schedules
The Writer magazine 114–15
Writers' and Artists' Yearbook (Pratchett) 38,
    61
writers' associations 114–15
writer's block 66–7
Writers' Guild 62
The Writer's Handbook (Turner) 61
writing the book
    avoiding distractions 65
    finding time 63–5
    overcoming 'blocks' 66–7
    plans and schedules 67, *68*
    postponing the task 66
    time allowances 4, 30–1, 33–5
    training courses 113–14
writing courses 113–14
writing schedules 3–5, 64–5
writing styles 85–90, 113–14
    experimentation and analyses 116–17,
        117